# Guidelines of Gross Anatomy

## Upper and Lower Limbs

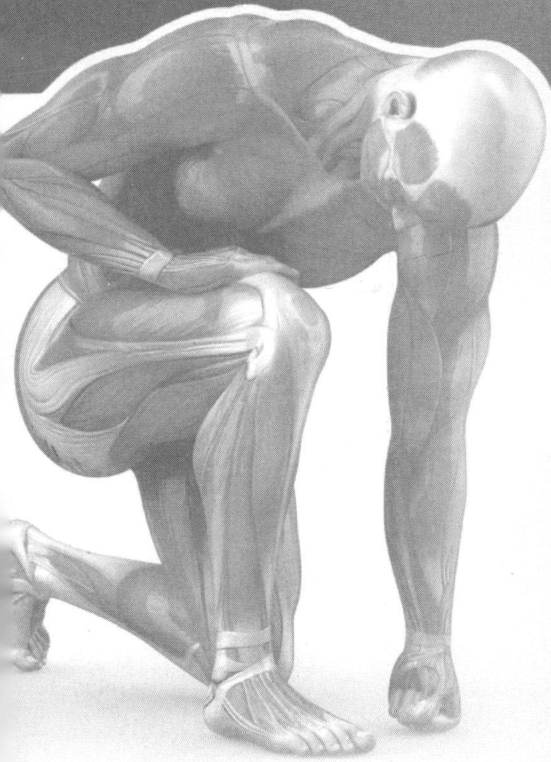

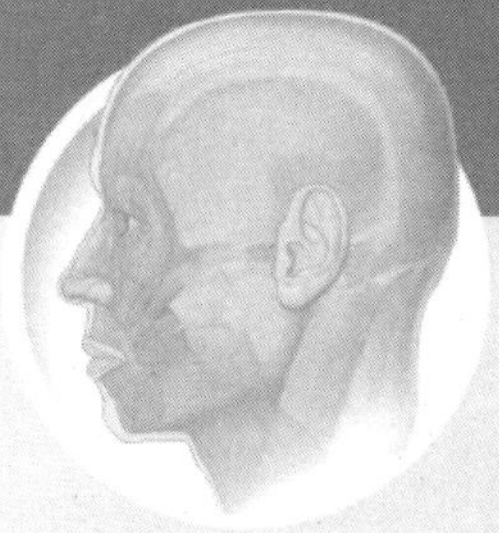

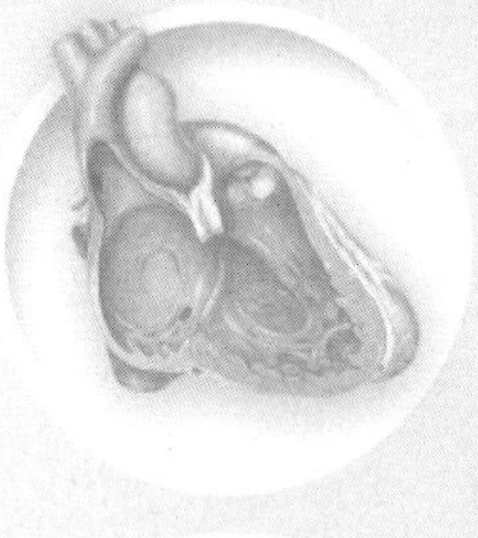

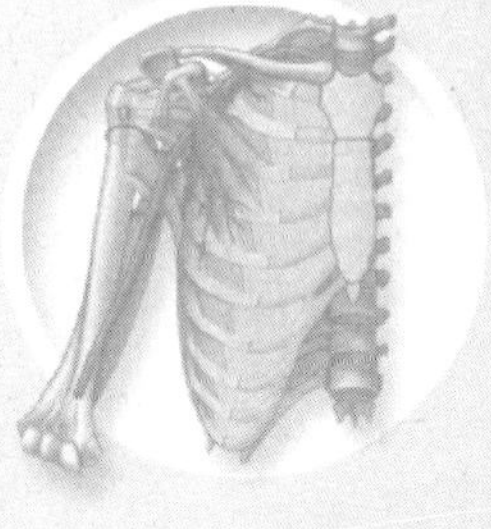

# GUIDELINES OF
# GROSS ANATOMY

## UPPER AND LOWER LIMB

**Wajid Hussain Barki**
MBBS, MCPS, M. Phil

**Paramount** Books (Pvt.) Ltd.
Karachi | Lahore | Islamabad | Hyderabad | Faisalabad | Peshawar | Abbottabad |

**Guidelines of Gross Anatomy**

by

Wajid Hussain Barki



First Edition .................. 2014

**Paramount** Books (Pvt.) Ltd.

152/O, Block-2, P.E.C.H.S., Karachi-75400. Tel: 34310030
Fax: 34553772, E-mail: info@paramountbooks.com.pk
Website: www.paramountbooks.com.pk

**ISBN: 978-969-637-015-4**

Printed in Pakistan

DEDICATED

TO

MY PARENTS AND FAMILY

# CONTENTS

## GENERAL ASPECTS


| | | |
|---|---|---|
| 01. | Introduction | 3 |
| 02. | Body tissues and structures | 9 |
| 03. | Bone and cartilage | 13 |
| 04. | Muscle | 21 |
| 05. | Joints | 29 |
| 06. | Circulatory system | 33 |
| 07. | Nervous system | 39 |
| 08. | Imaging techniques | 49 |
| 09. | SEQs | 53 |


## UPPER LIMB


| | | |
|---|---|---|
| 10. | Pectoral girdle | 57 |
| 11. | Shoulder | 71 |
| 12. | Axilla and breast | 81 |
| 13. | The arm | 99 |
| 14. | The forearm | 111 |
| 15. | The wrist and hand | 127 |
| 16. | Miscellaneous | 139 |
| 17. | SEQs | 147 |


## LOWER LIMB


| | | |
|---|---|---|
| 18. | Thigh | 151 |
| 19. | Gluteal region | 165 |
| 20. | Popliteal fossa and knee | 179 |
| 21. | The leg | 191 |
| 22. | The foot | 201 |
| 23. | Miscellaneous | 215 |
| 24. | SEQs | 223 |
| | Index | 225 |

# PREFACE

The aim of writing this book is to provide conceptual guidelines on the subject of anatomy, making it easy to understand, easy to remember, and easy to reproduce when required.

A very firm and consistent drive of my friends and the publisher kept me on the track and after four years of tedious work, this book has emerged in its final shape.

This book will prove to be a pleasant addition in the pool of medical books. The style and text of this book is different from other books. It is a student friendly version of gross anatomy. The concepts and descriptions have been explained in a simple and understandable way. Due emphases have been given to include all the essential topics of undergraduate syllabus and curriculum. SEQs from the previous professional examinations have been specifically included at the end of each section. It will help students become familiar with the format of the theory examination and will be helpful in self-assessment as well.

Further volumes of this book are in the pipeline and will be published in due course of time. Your feedback and suggestions will be welcomed and appreciated. It will help me to improve the next edition.

**Wajid Hussain Barki**

May, 2014

# ACKNOWLEDGEMENTS

I am highly indebted to my friends and fellow professionals who supported me while I was working on the manuscript of this book. I am especially grateful to Zainul Abedin, Director Paramount Books (Pvt.) Ltd. for his continuous, sincere and unlimited support throughout the entire period of publishing.

I must thank all those at Paramount Books who assisted in the publication of this book especially Asfiya Aziz, Manager Publishing, Dilshad Alam and Shoaib Ansari who worked on the title, format and graphics of this book with new ideas.

# SECTION 1

# GENERAL ASPECTS

## CONTENTS


| | | |
|---|---|---|
| 1 | Introduction | 3 |
| 2 | Body tissues and structures | 9 |
| 3 | Bone and cartilage | 13 |
| 4 | Muscle | 21 |
| 5 | Joints | 29 |
| 6 | Circulatory system | 33 |
| 7 | Nervous system | 39 |
| 8 | Imaging techniques | 49 |
| 9 | SEQs | 53 |

Chapter

# 1 INTRODUCTION

**ANATOMY** is defined as a branch of medical science which deals with the study of the structure of human body.

## BRANCHES OF ANATOMY

### 1. Gross Anatomy or Macroanatomy

It is defined as the study of the structures of living organisms that are visible to the naked eye. It is further subdivided into the follwoing.

a. ***General anatomy*** deals with the general aspects of the anatomy e.g. classification of muscles, bones and joints.

b. ***Regional anatomy*** explains the anatomy on the basis of different regions of the body e.g. head and neck, abdomen and thorax. Sometimes sub-regions like pectoral region, gluteal region, and parotid region may also be described on the same basis.

c. ***Systemic anatomy*** deals with the study of various parts, organs, and structures systematically e.g. nervous system, reproductive system, and GIT.

d. ***Surface anatomy*** deals with the recognition and identification of various structures in an individual externally just by inspection and palpation with reference to different established landmarks and imaginary planes of the body e.g. sternal notch, radial artery or surface anatomy of the kidneys.

### 2. Histology or Microanatomy

It is a branch of anatomy which deals with the study of fine details of body structures with the help of a microscope.

### 3. Embryology or Developmental Anatomy

It deals with all those processes and changes through which cells, tissues, organs and the body as a whole pass from fertilization to the birth and growth of the offspring. It includes:

a. ***Prenatal development:*** Development in the uterus of a mother before birth is called as intrauterine development.

b. ***Postnatal development:*** Development of an offspring which continues after birth leading to complete formation of an organ or structure until adulthood.

### 4. Other Branches of Anatomy

a. ***Applied anatomy*** is defined as anatomy applied to the diagnosis and treatment.

b. ***Comparative anatomy*** deals with the comparison of the structures of different species of animals with one another.

c. ***Radiological anatomy*** is the study of the anatomy of tissues based on their visualization on X-ray films.

d. ***Physiological or functional anatomy*** is the study of the structural details of organs with respect to their normal functions.

e. ***Investigative anatomy*** deals with different methods and techniques to explore the structural details of the human body to find or rule out any pathological lesion. It includes CT-scan, MRI, ultrasonography, angiography, gastroscopy, bronchoscopy and IVP (intravenous pyelography) etc.

## STRUCTURAL ORGANIZATION OF HUMAN BODY

The human body is composed of living matter called ***protoplasm***. This living matter constitutes the four basic levels of structural organization of the human body. These levels are:

### 1. Cell

A mass of protoplasm consisting of a nucleus and cytoplasm, bounded by a cell membrane is called a cell. Cells constitute the basic living units of structures and functions of an organization e.g. a neuron, hepatocyte, nephron or an osteocyte etc.

### 2. Tissue

It is a group of many similar cells that performs a specific function. There are four basic tissues of the body:

a. Epithelium

b. Connective tissue
c. Muscular tissue
d. Nervous tissue

### 3. Organ

An organ is a collection of two or more types of tissues that work together and perform a specific function e.g. kidney, liver, lung, heart, eye, and ear.

### 4. System or Organ System

It is a group of organs that work together and perform a specialized major function in the body e.g. nervous system, cardiovascular system, digestive, and urinary system etc.

All the systems of the body are coordinated and integrated with the constituent parts of their own system and with the other systems as well.

## ANATOMICAL POSITION

**Anatomical Position** is defined as the position of an individual in which he/she is

- standing erect,
- with arms by the sides,
- palms facing forwards,
- feet together,
- eyes looking straight.

Structures in the body are described in terms of their anatomical position.

## ANATOMICAL PLANES

These are imaginary planes used to facilitate the description of the anatomical relations and location. The major anatomical planes are as under.

### 1. Median Plane

It is a plane that divides the body vertically along the midline into two equal and symmetrical halves (right and left half). It is also known as midsagittal plane.

### 2. Sagittal Plane

Any vertical plane parallel to the median plane is called as sagittal plane. It divides the body into two unequal and asymmetrical halves.

### 3. Coronal Plane

Any plane passing longitudinally through the body from side to side at right angle to the median plane. It is also known as frontal plane.

### 4. Transverse or Horizontal Plane

In this plane, the body is divided into an upper and a lower part horizontally. They are at right angle to the medial, sagittal or coronal planes.

### 5. Axial Plane

Any plane parallel to the long axis of body (or a structure) is called an axial plane.

## ANATOMICAL TERMS AND POSITIONS

**Table 1-1: Terms of Anatomical Positions**

| Terms | Description |
|---|---|
| Anterior | Nearer the front of the body |
| Posterior | Nearer the back |
| Ventral | Analogue of anterior used in the trunk |
| Dorsal | Analogue of posterior used in the trunk |
| Medial | Nearer the median plane |
| Lateral | Away from the median plane |
| Superior | Towards the head |
| Inferior | Towards the tail |
| Cephalic | Analogue of superior |
| Caudal | Analogue of inferior |
| Superficial | Nearer the skin, used when direction is of no importance |

| | |
|---|---|
| Deep | Further from skin, used when direction is of no importance |
| External | Nearer the surface in any direction |
| Internal | Deep inward from the surface in any direction |
| Proximal | Nearer to, indicates the relative distance from the root of an organ or structure |
| Distal | Further from, indicates the relative distance from the root of an organ or structure |
| Palmar | Replaces anterior in hand |
| Plantar | Replaces inferior in foot |
| Cranial | Towards the head |
| Rostral | Situated toward a rostrum or toward the beak (oral and nasal region) |
| Radial or Fibular | Synonyms of lateral in forearm and leg |
| Ulnar or Tibial | Synonyms of medial in forearm and leg |

**Table 1-2: Terms of Movements**

| Movement | Description |
|---|---|
| Flexion | Folding or bending anteriorly. This movement occurs in sagittal plane. |
| Extension | Straightening or bending posteriorly. This movement also occur in sagittal plane. |
| Lateral flexion | Movement of the trunk (bending laterally) in the coronal plane |
| Adduction | Movement towards the median plane. This movement occurs in the coronal plane. |
| Abduction | Movement away from the median plane. This movement also occurs in the coronal plane. |
| Medial rotation | Inward movement of the anterior surface of a body part around its own longitudinal axis |
| Lateral rotation | Outward movement of the anterior surface of a body part around its own longitudinal axis |

| | |
|---|---|
| Circumd-uction | Showing all the movements successively i.e., flexion, extension, adduction, abduction, and rotation of a body part |
| Supination | The radius and ulna remain parallel and the palm of the hand faces anteriorly without any rotation. |
| Pronation | The radius and ulna rotate to overlap each other and the palm of the hand faces posteriorly without any rotation at the shoulder joint. |
| Opposition | To touch and oppose another body part e.g. thumb and index finger |
| Reposition | Reversal of opposition so that the body part returns to anatomical position |
| Inversion | Movement that turns the sole of the foot inward i.e., the individual stands on the lateral border of the foot |
| Eversion | Movement that turns the sole of the foot outward i.e., the individual stands on the medial border of the foot |
| Plantar-flexion | Movement of the foot towards the sole |
| Dorsiflexion | Movement of the foot towards the dorsum |
| Protraction | Forward movement of a body part |
| Retraction | Backward movement of an already forwarded placed body part |
| Elevation | Raising a body part |
| Depression | Lowering a body part |

**Table 1-3: Terms of Laterality**

| Movement | Description |
|---|---|
| Unilateral | Refers to one side of the body |
| Bilateral | Refers to both sides of the body (i.e., right and left) |
| Ipsilateral | Refers to the same side of the body |
| Contralateral | Refers to the opposite side of the body |
| Invagination | Intrusion of a part of the body into a hollow organ or a cavity |
| Evagination | Protrusion of a body part |

# Chapter 2 BODY TISSUES AND STRUCTURES

**Human** body is covered in different layers externally and internally e.g. skin, fascia, mucous and serous membranes. The connective tissues e.g. tendons and ligaments provide support and attachments to body organs. These structures, therefore, need a brief description.

## SKIN

Skin is the outermost covering of the body. It is the largest organ of the body. It consists of two layers:

1. Superficial layer or ***Epidermis***
2. Deep layer or ***Dermis***

The appendages of skin include Hair, Nails, Sweat, and Sebaceous glands. The thickness of skin varies from 0.5-3.0 mm and the total surface area in an average individual is 1.5-2.0 square meters. Skin performs the important function of protection, absorption, excretion, temperature regulation, synthesis of vitamin D and acts as a receptor for different sensations. It prevents the body both from hydration and dehydration because of its water proof property.

### Superficial Fascia

This layer lies just beneath the skin and is also called as *hypodermis* or *subcutaneous tissue*. It consists of loose areolar connective tissue. It is of variable thickness and fat content at different regions of the body. It is particularly dense in the scalp, palms, and soles. It is thinnest in the eyelids, and nipples. It is most distinct on the abdominal wall. The major function of the superficial fascia is to connect the skin with the deep fascia and bones. However, it also acts as a space filling and padding structure and is a site for the storage of fat. The fat is an insulating layer and accounts for the increased tolerance of cold in females.

## Deep Fascia

It is a membrane like structure of fibrous tissue, which wraps the body wall and the limbs. It is also of variable thickness and may be absent at certain regions like face. Its function at different anatomical planes and regions is different. Major functions of the deep fascia are as follows.

- It acts as an investing layer at certain regions of the body.
- It encloses neurovascular bundles, muscles and glands.
- It forms laminae of intermuscular septums.
- At certain locations it thickens to form bands of extensor and flexor retinaculae.
- It also forms fibrous sheaths on the fingers and toes.

## Ligament

Ligaments are structures composed of regular dense connective tissue. They mostly undergo stress and strains. They are attached at the ends of the bones and play very important role in the stability of joints. Ligaments are mostly rigid but flexible but not stretchable, however, ligamentum nuchae and ligamentum flava are exceptions due to the presence of a protein *elastin*.

## Tendon

Tendons are structures of regular dense connective tissue mainly the collagen fibers. They attach the muscles to bones. They are usually cylindrical in shape but sometimes it becomes flattened to form *aponeurosis*. It is estimated that 1 $cm^2$ of a tendon can support 1000kg weight.

## Synovial Sheath

These are the fibrous sheaths enveloping the tendons at the regions of friction. A synovial sheath consists of two layers:

1. The *parietal layer* is firmly adherent to the surrounding structures.
2. The *visceral layer* is fixed to the tendon.

They facilitate the gliding movements of the tendons between the two layers by lubricating them with the synovial fluid.

## Mucous Membrane

It is defined as the lining of internal body surface or a cavity which communicates externally. There are three components of mucous membrane:

a. *Epithelium:* It varies from region to region and system to system.
b. *Lamina propria:* It consists of connective tissue and is of variable thickness.
c. *Muscularis mucosae:* It consists of smooth muscle fibers and may be thin or even absent at some locations.

### Serous Membrane

It is the lining of a closed body cavity e.g. pericardial, pleural and peritoneal cavity. It is usually covered by a single layer of epithelium called as *mesothelium.* It consists of the following two layers:

1. *Parietal layer* is adherent to the wall of the cavity.
2. *Visceral layer* directly covers the organ or contents of the cavity.

## CLINICAL AND APPLIED INTEGRATION

### Estimation of Surface Area

The proportionate surface area of skin over different regions of the body is estimated by the *'rule of nines'*. According to this rule the approximate surface area of skin overlying the head is 9%, upper limb 9%, lower limb 18%, thorax 18% and abdomen 18%. This is a useful guide in assessing the surface area of skin for replacement of fluid loss from the body in cases of burns.

### Tension Lines

These lines were also described by Langer as *cleavage lines*. These are due to the patterns of collagen fibers in the dermis of the skin. Skin creases (*flexor lines*) and wrinkles of aging, run parallel to tension lines. Incisions made along skin tension lines heal with minimal scarring and are, therefore, used for cosmetic surgery.

### Sprains

Injury to the ligaments leading to intractable pain and restricting the movements of the affected part e.g. Injury by jumping or running on an uneven ground is called as sprain. Some of the fibers of the ligaments are damaged but the continuity remains intact. Mostly athletes and sportsmen are victims of this kind of injuries.

Chapter

# 3 BONE AND CARTILAGE

**Bone** is a type of vascularized dense connective tissue with cells embedded in a matrix composed of organic materials, (mainly collagen fibers) and inorganic salts, (mainly calcium and phosphate). Mineralization of the bone matrix is responsible for the hardness of the bone. Bony tissue is also known as *osseous tissue*.

## TYPES OF BONES

1. **Compact (Haversian) bone** consists of haversian system or osteons. It is very hard and dense.
2. **Spongy (Cancellous) bone** consists of an irregular meshwork of intercommunicating bony trabeculae and, therefore, presents an interwoven pattern of bony tissues.

### Parts of a Long Bone

1. Shaft ..............Diaphysis
2. Neck..............Metaphysis (junction of epiphysis and diaphysis)
3. Proximal (upper) end } *Epiphysis*
4. Distal (lower) end } *Epiphysis*

## REGIONAL DISTRIBUTION OF BONES

The distribution of bones in different regions of the body is as under:

1. Appendicular bones: 126
2. Axial bones: 80

**Table 3-1: Appendicular Bones**

| Bones of upper limb | No. of bones | Bones of lower limb | No. of bones |
|---|---|---|---|
| Shoulder girdle | 04 | Hip girdle | 02 |
| | | Thigh | 02 |
| Upper arm | 02 | Knee | 02 |
| Forearm | 04 | Leg | 04 |
| Wrist (carpal) | 16 | Ankle (tarsal) | 14 |
| Hand (metacarpal) | 10 | Foot (metatarsal) | 10 |
| Phalanges | 28 | Toes | 28 |
| **Total** | **64** | **Total** | **62** |

**Table 3-2: Axial Bones**

| Region | No. of bones |
|---|---|
| Skull | 22 |
| Ear (ossicles) | 06 |
| Hyoid | 01 |
| Vertebral column | 26 |
| Ribs | 24 |
| Sternum | 01 |
| **Total** | **80** |

## CLASSIFICATION OF BONES

1. Regional Classification

    a. **Axial bones** include the skull, vertebral column, and bones of the thorax etc.

    b. **Appendicular bones** include bones of upper and lower limbs.

## 2. Architectural Classification

a. **Compact** e.g. shaft of long bones

b. **Spongy** e.g. diploë of skull

## 3. Classification According to Size and Shape

a. **Long bones** e.g. humerus, ulna, femur, metacarpal and metatarsal bones

b. **Short bones** e.g. carpal bones, tarsal bones etc.

c. **Flat bones** e.g. ribs, sternum, scapulae, and bones of skull vault

d. **Irregular bones** e.g. hip bones, sphenoid, temporal, and zygomatic bones etc

e. **Sesamoid bones** e.g. patella

f. **Accessory bones** e.g. cervical rib, wormian bones, os trigonum tarsi (also called supernumery bone), and rider's bones (also called heterotropic bones). These bones develop in the adductor muscles of horse riders.

g. **Pneumatic bones** e.g. ethmoid, maxilla, sphenoid bones

## 4. Embryological Classification

a. **Membranous bones:** These bones develop by the intramembranous method of osteogenesis e.g. flat bones of skull and bones of the face (nasal bones, maxilla, and zygotic bones) and clavicle of the shoulder girdle.

b. **Cartilaginous bones:** These bones develop by the intracartilagenous method of osteogenesis e.g. long bones, ribs and vertebrae, etc.

c. **Membrano-cartilaginous bones:** The development of these bones is partially intramembranous and partially intracartilagenous e.g. mandible, occipital, temporal and sphenoid bones etc.

## 5. Evolutionary Classification

a. **Exoskeleton** e.g. enamel of teeth

b. **Endoskeleton:** All other bones

**Table 3-3: Description of Impressions and Markings on a Bone**

| | |
|---|---|
| Head | A rounded articular surface at the upper extremity (usually connected by a neck) |
| Capitulum | A small eminence on a bone by which it articulates with another bone |
| Trochlea | A pulley shaped structure |
| Condyle | A rounded, knuckle-like articular area or a rounded projection |
| Facet | A small smooth and flat surface on a bone |
| Fossa | A hollow or depressed area |
| Process | A prominence or a projection |
| Trochanter | A large blunt process (may be flat or conical) |
| Tuberosity | A rounded elevation or protuberance |
| Tubercle | A small rounded eminence |
| Malleolus | A small rounded process or protuberance |
| Epicondyle | An eminence or projection on or above a condyle |
| Spine | Slender, thorn-like pointed process |
| Styloid | Long and pointed resembling a pillar |
| Hamulus | A projection resembling a hook |
| Line | A strip, streak or a narrow ridge |
| Crest | A prominent ridge especially one surrounding a bone or its border |
| Fovea | A small pit or depression |
| Notch | An indentation on the edge of a bone |
| Fissure | A narrow cleft or deep groove |
| Foramen | A natural opening or passage |
| Meatus | An opening or passage |
| Groove | A narrow linear hollow or depression |
| Sulcus | Trench or furrow like depression |
| Hiatus | A gap or a cleft |

## BLOOD SUPPLY OF LONG BONES

### 1. Arterial Supply

a. **Nutrient arteries:** These arteries pass into the medullary cavity and divide into ascending and descending branches called *medullary arteries*. Some of the terminal branches anastomose with the branches of metaphyseal arteries.

b. **Metaphyseal arteries:** These are direct branches of major regional arteries. The branches anastomose with the terminal branches of medullary arteries.

c. **Epiphyseal arteries:** These are derived from the network of anastomosis formed around the joint by the branches of surrounding major arteries. They form arterial arches at each bone end.

d. **Periosteal arteries:** These are derived from the muscular arteries of those muscles which are attached to the bone.

### 2. Venous Drainage

a. **In the medullary cavity:** *Central Venous Sinus* (located in the center of medullary cavity) receives blood from:

  i. The meshwork of medullary sinusoids fed by central branches of medullary arteries;

  ii. End arterial loops formed by the terminal branches of the medullary arteries;

  iii. Central Venous Sinus drains blood into the diaphyseal vein.

b. **In the periosteum:** Periosteal venous plexus and periosteal veins receive blood from the cortical capillaries and drain this blood into the muscular veins.

## FUNCTIONS OF THE BONES

1. Provide characteristic and peculiar shape to an individual
2. Support and locomotion e.g. sitting, walking, running, climbing and jumping
3. Protection of vital organs e.g. skull and thoracic cage protecting the brain and heart

4. Surface for attachment of muscles, ligaments, and tendons
5. Site for the formation of new blood cells *(erythropoiesis)*
6. Assist in hearing e.g. ear ossicles
7. Stores of calcium and phosphorus
8. Chief sites for reticuloendothelial system of the body
9. Help in respiration e.g. ribs and sternum
10. Facilitate chewing e.g. mandible and maxilla along with teeth
11. Used as an index to assess the age of an individual
12. Detoxification and deposition centers for certain elements e.g. lead, arsenic, fluorine, and radium and for toxins and drugs like tetracyclines

## CLASSIFICATION OF CARTILAGES

There are three types of cartilages:

1. Hyaline cartilage
2. Fibrocartilage
3. Elastic cartilage

**Table 3-4: General Features of Cartilages**

| S. No. | Features | Hyaline Cartilage | Fibrocartilage | Elastic Cartilage |
|---|---|---|---|---|
| 1. | Appearance and Nature | • Translucent (glassy)<br>• Rigid and strong | • Resilient<br>• Pliable | • Flexible<br>• Elastic |
| 2. | Function | Support | • Resists tension<br>• Absorbs shock | • Allows distortion<br>• Provides flexibility |

| | | | | |
|---|---|---|---|---|
| 3. | Distribution | • Articular cartilages<br>• Trachea<br>• Bronchi<br>• Costal cartilages<br>• Nasal septum etc. | • Intervertebral discs labrum glenoidale<br>• Labrum acetabulare<br>• Intra-articular discs<br>• Menisci etc. | • Pinna<br>• Auditory tube<br>• Epiglottis |

## CLINICAL AND APPLIED INTEGRATION

### Fracture

It is defined as a break in the continuity (or rupture) of a bone. Fractures are of two types:

1. *Simple* or closed fractures in which the fragments of the bone do not communicate externally.
2. *Compound* or open in which the fracture fragments communicate externally through a wound.

In *Green stick fractures*, the fractured segments of the bone never separate, instead there is bowing of the bone. This type of a fracture occurs in children.

*Spontaneous fractures* may be seen in those who are suffering from bone diseases like tumours of the bones, or error in the calcium metabolism.

### Osteoporosis

Abnormal rarefaction of bone is called as osteoporosis. The organic and inorganic components of bone decrease during the aging process. The bones become brittle and fracture easily. Females are more prone to osteoporosis after the onset of menopause.

### Osteomalacia

This condition is caused by the inadequate or delayed mineralization of osteoid in the mature bone. Severe bone pain and multiple fractures are the common presentations. Liver diseases and tumours usually induce this condition. This condition is confined to adults only. The equivalent of osteomalacia in children is called as *rickets.*

## Osteomyelitis

It is the chronic (long standing) inflammation of the bones. It may be localized or generalized. The cause is usually an infection of the bone by some pyogenic organism. Tuberculosis is one of the most common causes of this disorder.

## Age Assesment

The age of an individual is determined by studying the ossification centers in bones. The evaluation of bone age is done by taking radiographs (X-rays) of different bones. The ossification centers are studied for:

1. Location and number of centers,
2. Time of appearance and
3. Fusion of these centers.

The bones are, therefore, used as a parameter of age assessment.

Chapter

# 4 MUSCLE

**Muscle** is a special type of connective tissue capable of contraction and relaxation. It, therefore, brings about the movements of a part or the body as a whole. Muscle being an organ constitutes the muscular system. A muscle cell or *myocyte* is also called as a *muscle fiber* because it is cylindrical in shape.

A muscle is defined as a collection of fascicles of muscle fibers (of any type) and also surrounded by connective tissue proper.

## TYPES OF MUSCULAR TISSUE

1. **Skeletal or striated muscle** shows rapid and unsustained contractions under the control of nervous system.
2. **Smooth muscle** is devoid of any type of striations. They show slow and sustained contractions. They are controlled by the autonomous nervous system.
3. **Cardiac muscle** is composed of cylindrical, branching, and anastomosing contractile cells. They show myogenic rhythmic contractions. However, their activity is modified by autonomic nervous system.

### Parts of a Skeletal Muscle

#### *1. Origin*

The part of a muscle which remains fixed during the muscle contraction.

#### *2. Belly or gaster*

The fleshy part of a muscle capable of contraction and relaxation.

### *3. Insertion*

The part which moves or brings about movements. It may be:

a. *Muscular* e.g. mylohyoid,

b. *Tendinous* e.g. deltoid,

c. *Aponeurotic* e.g. Palmaris longus,

d. *Tendino-aponeurotic* i.e. dual e.g. biceps brachii.

## CLASSIFICATION OF SKELETAL MUSCLES

### Classification on the Basis of Fiber Architecture

1. **Muscles with fibers parallel to the line of pull**
   a. ***Strap-like muscles:*** e.g. Sartorius, sternohyoid, and sternothyroid
   b. ***Quadrilateral muscles:*** e.g. pronator quadratus and thyrohyoid
   c. ***Fusiform muscles:*** e.g. biceps brachii
2. **Muscles with fibers oblique to the line of pull**
   a. ***Triangular muscles:*** e.g. deltoid, Trapezius, and temporalis
   b. ***Pennate muscles:***
      - Unipennate muscles e.g. peroneus tertius and flexor policis longus
      - Bipennate muscles e.g. rectus femoris, dorsal interossei (of hand and foot)
      - Multipennate muscles e.g. subscapularis and deltoid muscle
   c. ***Radial muscle:*** also called as circumpennate muscle e.g. tibialis anterior
3. **Spiral muscles:** e.g. latissimus dorsi etc.
4. **Cruciate muscles** e.g. masseter and sternocleidomastoid
5. **Circular (or sphincteral) muscles** e.g. orbicularis oculi and orbicularis oris

### Classification on the Basis of Group Action

1. **Agonist:** Muscles constantly active in the initiation and

maintenance of a movement. These muscles are also called *prime movers*.

2. **Antagonist:** Muscles acting against the action of the agonists
3. **Synergists:** Muscles preventing the unwanted movements during the action of an agonist
4. **Fixators:** Muscles which stabilize one attached and of a muscle so that the other end may move

Movements are the result of the coordinated activity of many muscles, sometimes assisted by gravity.

### *Contraction of muscles*

There are three types of contractions in skeletal muscles.

1. **Reflex contraction:** Involuntary contraction of the diaphragm muscles and skeletal muscle tendon leading to a jerk (e.g. knee jerk, ankle jerk)
2. **Tonic contraction:** The continuous, conscious and a normal degree of contraction of a skeletal muscle giving it some firmness for maintaining body posture is called tonic contraction or muscle tone. It is lost during sleep and unconsciousness.
3. **Phasic contraction:** It is the active and wilful contraction of a skeletal muscle. It is of two types:
    a. ***Isotonic contraction***
        i. Concentric contraction: when movement occurs as a result of shortening of a muscle e.g. agonists
        ii. Eccentric contraction: when a contracting muscle increases in length due to gradual relaxation of its fibers e.g. antagonists
    b. ***Isometric contraction:*** The muscle tension rises above the tonic level without any movement or increase in muscle length.

## Functional Classification

1. **Voluntary muscles**

    Constitute 43% of total body weight

    a. Skeletal muscles:
        - All skeletal muscles
        - Muscles of upper third of esophagus

- Respiratory muscles
- Muscles of mastication and facial expression

b. Smooth muscles:

Ciliary body muscles (of accommodation)

2. **Involuntary muscles**
   a. Smooth muscles of GIT, genital, urinary system
   b. Muscles of pharynx, larynx
   c. Muscles of lower 2/3 of esophagus
   d. Iris muscles
   e. Arrector pilorum
   f. Trachealis muscle
   g. Muscles in the walls of blood vessels
   h. Muscles around the acini of some glands
   i. Dartos muscle in the hypodermis of scrotum
3. **Cardiac muscles**

   Control of contraction in cardiac muscle is inherent myogenic activity. Heart starts beating in the third week of intrauterine life when the nervous system is in the process of early differentiation.

## Classification According to the Amount of Myoglobin

1. **Red muscle fiber:** They contain relatively abundant myoglobin and mitochondria. The sarcoplasm of red muscle fiber contains high content of myoglobin (which gives it red colour). The diameter of these fibers is small. They are also called *slow twitch fibers* because they are able for prolonged and steady contraction e.g. soleus, erector spinae.
2. **White muscle fiber:** They have longer diameter, less myoglobin, and few mitochondria. They are able to contract more rapidly but fatigue very quickly; hence are called as *fast twitch fibers* e.g. Gastrocnemius, muscles of the eye and hand.
3. **Intermediate muscle fiber:** The intermediate fibers are a mixture of red and white muscle fibers and so exhibit both fast and slow twitch activity.

The proportions of these three types of skeletal muscle fibers vary from muscle to muscle and even within various regions of a particular muscle.

## Classification According to the Phylogenetic History

1. **Somatic muscles** develop from myotomes.
   a. ***Somatic axial muscles*** e.g. trunk and extraocular muscles
   b. ***Somatic appendicular*** e.g. muscles of the limbs
2. **Visceral muscles**
   a. ***Visceral pharyngeal muscles*** develop from the mesenchyme of pharyngeal apparatus e.g.
      i. tensor tympani
      ii. stapedius
      iii. muscles of mastication
   b. ***Visceral smooth muscles*** develop from the mesenchyme surrounding the endodermal gut tube e.g. smooth muscles of stomach, intestine, and urinary bladder.

# FUNCTIONS OF MUSCLES

## 1. Skeletal Muscle

a. Maintenance of body posture
b. Locomotion
c. Production of heat
d. Pumping of venous blood towards the heart
e. Exhibition of expressions e.g. sorrow, grief, and joy etc.

## 2. Smooth Muscle

a. Pushing of food through GIT
b. Excretion of the waste through GIT and urinary bladder
c. Expulsion of the fetus from the uterus (delivery) at the end of gestation period
d. Hemostasis by compressing the bleeding vessels

## 3. Cardiac Muscle

a. Beating of the heart
b. Rhythmicity of the heart by synchronous contraction of muscle fibers

## INNERVATION OF SKELETAL MUSCLE

### Motor Supply

1. **Alpha efferent** comprising myelinated axons. These are extrafusal fibers of large size. They terminate at the neuromuscular junctions (also called as *motor end plate*). An α-axon supplying a muscle fiber or a group of muscle fibers constitutes a *motor unit*.
2. **Gamma efferent** comprises thin intrafusal fibers located within the muscle spindle. They are also myelinated but lose the myelin sheath as they enter into the muscle spindle. They are concerned with the contraction of the muscle.

### Sensory Supply

1. **Muscle spindle** also consists of intrafusal fibers. Intrafusal fibers are thin modified skeletal muscle fibers located within the bag of connective tissues and has lost cross striations. Here the sensory receptors give origin to two types of afferent fibers:
   a. Annulospiral fibers
   b. Flower spray fibers

   These fibers become myelinated after they emerge from the muscle spindle. They are concerned with the position and vibration sense.
2. **Free nerve endings** are very fine non-myelinated nerve fibers concerned with the sensation of pain. They are located in the sheath of connective tissues which is covering the muscle.

## PRE-AXIAL AND POST-AXIAL BORDERS

Each limb is divided into a *flexor* and an *extensor* compartment. Both the compartments embryologically meet at pre-axial and post-axial borders. These borders in the limbs are represented by the following structures:

### Upper Limb

Pre-axial border is represented by the cephalic vein.

Post-axial border is represented by the basalic vein.

## Lower Limb

Pre-axial border is represented by the great saphenous vein.

Post-axial border is represented by the small saphenous vein.

## CLINICAL AND APPLIED INTEGRATION

### Muscle Tear (Pulled Muscle or Muscle Spasm)

Skeletal muscles have limited ability to lengthen. Normally *muscles cannot elongate more than one third of the resting length*. If a muscle is forced to elongate excessively, muscle tears occur due to the eccentric contraction of the muscle. It usually occurs due to the sudden involuntary and violent contraction. This condition is known as muscle strain and the muscle or group of muscles involved is called '*pulled muscle*'. Weight lifters and athletes usually sustain these injuries.

### Muscle Paralysis and Muscle Paresis

When the nerve supplying a skeletal muscle is damaged as a result of an injury or disease, it loses its ability to contract. This condition is known as paralysis or palsy. *Facial palsy* is the classical example in which muscles of the facial expressions are paralyzed due to the damage to facial nerve. Paralysis of the muscles of one half (right or left) of the body is called as *hemiplegia*. The term *paraplegia* implies paralysis of the lower half of the body whereas paralysis of the lower half of one side is known as *hemiparaplegia*. *Quadriplegia* is the paralysis of the muscles of all four limbs. Partial paralysis or partial loss of muscle power i.e., loss of the ability to contract, is called as muscle *paresis*. These conditions occur due to injury to the nerves or due to some neuronal disorder e.g. hemorrhage or a clot interfering with the blood supply of higher centers.

# Chapter 5 JOINTS

**Joint** is defined as a union between two or more bones or cartilages. Joints exhibit a variety of forms and functions. A joint is also called as an *articulation*.

## CLASSIFICATION OF JOINTS

1. Joints without a cavity or solid joints **Synarthroses**
2. Joints with a cavity Synovial joints or **Diarthroses**

### 1. Synarthroses

#### *a. Fibrous joints*

i. **Sutural joints**
   - Serrate sutures
   - Denticulate sutures
   - Squamous sutures
   - Plain sutures
   - Schindylesis

ii. **Syndemoses**

iii. **Gomphoses**

#### *b. Cartilaginous joints*

i. **Synchondroses** (Primary Cartilaginous Joints)

ii. **Symphyses** (Secondary Cartilaginous Joints)

### 2. Diarthroses or Synovial Joints

#### a. Classification According to the Complexity of Form

i. **Simple joints** e.g. shoulder joint, interphalangeal joints

ii. **Compound joints** e.g. elbow joint

iii. **Complex joints** e.g. knee joint and sternoclavicular joint

## b. Classification According to the Degree of Freedom of movements

i. **Uniaxial** e.g. interphalangeal joints

ii. **Biaxial** e.g. wrist joint

iii. **Multiaxial** e.g. shoulder joint

## c. Classification According to the Shape/Arrangement of the Articulating Surfaces

i. **Plane joints** e.g. intermetatarsal joints

ii. **Hinge joints** e.g. elbow joint

iii. **Pivot joints** e.g. superior radioulnar joint

iv. **Bicondylar joints** e.g. knee joint, temporomandibular joint

v. **Ellipsoid joints** e.g. wrist joint

vi. **Sellar or saddle joints** e.g. ankle joint

vii. **Spheroidal or ball and socket joints** e.g. hip joint, shoulder joint

## Characteristics of Synovial Joints

Typical synovial joints are characterized by six features.

1. Bone ends taking part are covered by hyaline cartilage.
2. Joint is surrounded by a capsule enclosing a joint cavity.
3. Joint cavity is internally lined by synovial membrane.
4. Joint is reinforced by ligaments.
5. It is capable of various degrees of movements.
6. The articular surfaces of atypical synovial joints are covered by fibrocartilage e.g. temporomandibular joint.

## Structural Components of Synovial Joints

### 1. *Fibrous capsule*

It surrounds and holds the bones together like a cuff but at the same time permits movements due to its pliable nature and laxity.

## 2. *Ligaments*

These are the fibrous bands of dense connective tissues which connect the adjacent bones of a joint. They provide strength and support to the joints. Ligaments may be:

a. ***Intracapsular*** e.g. cruciate ligaments of knee joint and ligament of head of femur, etc.

b. ***Extracapsular*** e.g. coracoclavicular, sacrotuberous ligaments etc.

c. ***Capsular ligaments*** due to the thickening of the joint capsule in the region of stress and strain e.g. radial and ulnar collateral ligaments, iliofemoral ligament, etc.

## 3. *Synovial membrane*

It is a highly vascular thin membrane which lines the inner surface of the fibrous capsule except the articular cartilage, articular discs and menisci. It takes part in the production and absorption of synovial fluid. It facilitates the joint movements and also shows phagocytic activity.

## 4. *Articular cartilage*

It is a hyaline type of cartilage which covers the articulating surfaces of the bones. It acts as a shock absorber. It is devoid of nerves and is avascular as well.

## 5. *Articular discs*

These are the pads of fibrocartilage which divide the joint cavity into complete or incomplete compartments e.g. temporomandibular and inferior radioulnar joints.

## 6. *Menisci*

It is a crescent shaped fibrocartilage interposed between the articulating surfaces e.g. medial and lateral menisci of knee joint.

## 7. *Labra*

This is a pliable ring of fibrocartilage attached to the rim of a bony socket increasing its depth e.g. labrum glenoidale and labrum acetabulum.

### 8. *Synovial fluid*

It is the transparent, viscid and shiny fluid present in the joint cavity. It provides nutrition and lubrication to the synovial joints.

## HILTON'S LAW OF NERVE SUPPLY OF JOINTS

This law states " *The motor nerve to a muscle tends to give a branch to the joint which the muscle moves as well as the skin overlying that joint.*"

## CLINICAL AND APPLIED INTEGRATION

### Dislocation of a Joint

Disruption or displacement of a bone or bones constituting a joint from their normal anatomical position is called as dislocation. The weakest joint prone to dislocation is the shoulder joint due to shallow glenoid cavity and lack of support inferiorly. However, congenital dislocation of hip joint in infants is also common.

### Osteoarthritis

It is a degenerative condition of old age characterized by pain, stiffness and difficulty in locomotion. It is caused by the degenerative changes in the articular cartilage affecting the mechanism of lubrication and its capability as shock absorber. Weight bearing joints like hip and knee joints are more affected.

Chapter

# 6 CIRCULATORY SYSTEM

**Circulatory** system comprises: (1) cardiovascular system and (2) lymphoid system. Cardiovascular system includes heart and blood vessels, whereas lymphoid system includes afferent and efferent lymphatic vessels and lymphoid organs. The chief function of the circulatory system is to maintain the homeostasis i.e., constancy of internal environment in the body and transportation of materials.

## CLASSIFICATION OF BLOOD VESSELS

### 1. Anatomical Classification

#### *a. Arteries*

Vessels that carry the blood away from the heart to different body parts, organs and structures, are called arteries.

i. **Elastic arteries** e.g. aorta, subclavian arteries, contain a large number of elastic fibers in the tunica media. They are also known as large arteries.

ii. **Muscular arteries** e.g. radial, ulnar, femoral arteries contain a large number of smooth muscles in the tunica media. These are *medium sized arteries* and are also known as *conducting vessels*.

#### *b. Arterioles*

These are the *small arteries* having a diameter of 0.2-0.4 mm and are responsible to regulate the blood pressure. Smaller arterioles are called as *terminal arterioles*. The smaller vessels, formed as a result of branching of arterioles, are called *metarterioles*.

***Preferential or thoroughfare channels***

In certain regions of the body metarterioles give rise to capillaries and then directly open into the venules. They act as low resistance channels. When the precapillary sphincters constrict, they provide substitute route to the flow of blood. They bypass the capillary beds in cases of reduced blood flow through them. They are most numerous in the skin, mesenteries and pinna.

### c. *Capillaries*

These are the microscopic vessels which connect the arterial and venous ends of circulation. An average length of a capillary is 0.75 mm and diameter of 7-9 mm. Capillaries are of three types:

i. **Continuous capillaries** do not have any pores or gaps in their walls. This type of vessels are found in brain, muscles and lungs.

ii. **Fenestrated capillaries** are characterized by the presence of pores in their walls. They are found in the kidneys, endocrine glands and intestines.

iii. **Sinusoidal capillaries** have larger lumen which is irregular and contain pores. They are found in liver, spleen and suprarenal glands.

### d. *Venules*

These are the vessels that collect venous blood from the capillaries or capillary plexuses and unite to form veins. There are three segments of a venule:

i. **Postcapillary venule:** A postcapillary venule is formed by the union of two or more capillaries. They mainly consist of endothelium and thin adventitia. The exchange of water solutes and leukocytes into the intercellular space takes place through these vessels. They are the important sites of inflammation.

ii. **Muscular venule:** They are formed by the union of postcapillary venules. They contain smooth muscles in the tunica media.

iii. **Collecting venule:** The muscular venules join to form collecting venules. They drain blood into veins.

### e. *Veins*

Veins are formed by the union of smaller veins or venules. The small veins constituting a large vein are called *tributaries.* Large veins especially those of the lower limb have the valves. Veins are further classified as:

i. **Small veins** include unnamed veins of the body.

ii. **Medium-sized veins** include named veins of the body e.g. cephalic vein, basalic vein, axillary vein, popliteal and great saphenous veins, etc.

iii. **Large veins** include superior and inferior venae cavae, common iliac veins, etc.

***Venae comitantes***

The major or named arteries lying in the deeper regions of the limbs are usually accompanied by a pair of veins, one on either side of that artery, called venae comitantes. They are given the name of the corresponding artery. They are connected with each other at many places.

## 2. Physiological Classification

### a. *Conducting vessels*

These comprise the large or elastic arteries. These include aorta, pulmonary trunk, common carotid, common iliac, and subclavian arteries.

### b. *Distribution vessels*

These are the medium-sized muscular arteries. These supply the individual organs and structures and divide into branches within the substance of that organ.

### c. *Resistance vessels*

This group includes arterioles and metarterioles. The lumen of these vessels is small but they have relatively thick walls. Due to this reason they are the source of peripheral resistance to the flow of blood.

### d. *Exchange vessels*

This group of vessels includes postcapillary venules, capillaries and sinusoids. They allow the exchange of substances between blood and tissue fluids. The walls of these vessels consist of endothelium only.

### e. *Reservoir or capacitance vessels*

These are large volume and low resistance vessels. Due to their ability to distend, they can accommodate large volumes of blood.

They include large sized venules, muscular and elastic veins. Usually 70% of the total blood volume remains in the pool of these vessels.

### *f. Shunts*

Shunts are the physiological bypass channels to regulate the flow of blood according to the body needs. These are usually found at the pre-capillary and pre-sinusoidal level.

## Anastomosis of Blood Vessels

It is defined as the free communication between the ends of arterioles and venules. There are three types of anastomoses which occur in human body:

### *1. Arterial anastomoses*

a. *End-to-end anastomosis* occurs between the right and left gastro-epiploic arteries.

b. *Transverse anastomosis* occurs between ulnar and radial arteries by means of a transverse link.

c. *Convergence anastomosis* occurs between right and left vertebral arteries which converge to form a single basilar artery.

### *2. Venous anastomoses*

It is a communication between the ends of veins or the tributaries of veins. Classical examples are:

a. Dorsal venous arch of hand and

b. Dorsal venous arch of foot.

### *3. Arteriovenous anastomoses*

These channels serve as a pathway for shunting the arterial blood directly into the venous blood. They regulate the local blood flow in specific regions of the body at the time of functional demands. They are found in the:

a. skin of fingertips, lips, nose and pinna,

b. mucosa of stomach and small intestine.

### *End arteries*

Those arteries which do not anastomose with their neighbour vessels are called as end arteries. They are usually the sole source of blood supply to a region. The blockage of such arteries is lethal and thus leads to cell death of the area of supply. Central artery of the retina is the classical example of an end artery. They are also found in the kidneys, brain, spleen, and mesenteries (vasa recta) etc.

## TYPES OF CIRCULATIONS

According to the route followed by the blood flow, the following types of circulations can be seen in the human body:

1. Systemic circulation
2. Pulmonary circulation
3. Portal circulation
4. Coronary circulation
5. Hypophyseal-hypothalamic circulation
6. Collateral circulation

## CLINICAL AND APPLIED INTEGRATION

### Varicose Veins

This is the condition characterized by the abnormal dilatation of the veins and is called as *varicosity*. The common cause is the incompetent valves of the affected veins. The superficial veins of the lower limb suffer more due to the failure of propulsion of blood towards heart side through these veins against the gravity. These veins become prominent, tortuous, and dilated due to pooling of blood. In long standing cases sometimes overlying skin may ulcerate.

### Atherosclerosis

This is the most common condition affecting the arteries. In this condition gradual *narrowing and hardening* of the vessels occurs due to the deposits in the vessel walls. These deposits are mostly calcium or fat in nature. Atherosclerosis may lead to *ischemia* of the area of supply by the affected vessel i.e., death of tissues due to lack of oxygen supply. The usual outcome of the ischemia of the heart tissues is *heart attack* due to the narrowing of the coronary vessels by the atherosclerosis.

## LYMPHOID SYSTEM

This system consists of:

1. Lymph vessels
    a. Afferent lymphatics
    b. Efferent lymphatics
2. Lymphoid organs

### Lymph Vessels

These are fine tubes that contain a clear fluid called as *lymph*. Lymph is collected from the tissues by a closed network of lymph capillaries which converge on the lymph nodes. From the lymph nodes it is finally drained in the blood stream. The vessels which carry the lymph to a node are called as *afferent lymphatics* and those which carry it away from a node are called as *efferent lymphatics*.

### Lymphoid Organs

Lymphoid organs include:

1. Lymph nodes
2. Spleen
3. Thymus
4. Tonsils:
    a. Palatine tonsils
    b. Lingual tonsils
    c. Pharyngeal tonsils
    d. Tubal tonsils

### CLINICAL AND APPLIED INTEGRATION

The significance of lymphoid system lies in:

1. The spread of diseases like bacterial infections,
2. Blockade of lymph channels leading to diseases like elephantiasis,
3. Spread of cancer,
4. Production of lymphocytes and initiation of immune reactions,
5. Participation in phagocytosis,
6. Removal of dead blood cells and
7. Filtration of blood and removal of toxins.

Chapter

# 7 NERVOUS SYSTEM

**Nervous** system is the co-ordination and integration center of the body for external and internal responses. All the body functions are centrally controlled and influenced by the nervous system.

## CLASSIFICATION OF NERVOUS SYSTEM

### 1. Central Nervous System

a. **Brain**
   i. Cerebrum
   ii. Cerebellum
   iii. Brain stem
      - Midbrain
      - Pons
      - Medulla oblongata

b. **Spinal cord**

### 2. Peripheral Nervous System

a. **Peripheral nerves**
   i. Spinal nerves
   ii. Cranial nerves

b. **Ganglia**
   i. Sensory or dorsal root ganglia
   ii. Autonomic ganglia

### 3. Autonomic Nervous System

a. Sympathetic nervous system
b. Parasympathetic nervous system

## Embryological Classification of Nervous System

### 1. Prosencephalon or Forebrain

a. **Telencephalon**
   i. Cerebrum
   ii. Limbic system
   iii. Basal nuclei

b. **Diencephalon**
   i. Thalamus
   ii. Hypothalamus
   iii. Metathalamus
   iv. Epithalamus
   v. Subthalamus

### 2. Mesencephalon or Midbrain

### 3. Rhombencephalon or Hindbrain

a. **Metencephalon**
   i. Pons
   ii. Cerebellum

b. **Mylencephalon**
   i. Medulla oblongata

### 4. Spinal Cord

Nervous system is made up of nervous tissues. There are three types of tissues which constitute the nervous system:

1. Nerve cells or *neurons*
2. Supporting cells or glial *tissues*
3. Connective tissue or *coverings*

## NEURON

Neuron is the structural and functional unit of nervous system. A neuron is a type of nervous tissue which is capable of excitability and conductivity.

### Parts of a Neuron

1. A cell body or *soma* which contains the nucleus
2. Short processes or *dendrites* which receive stimuli or impulses
3. A long process or an *axon* which conducts the impulses

### Morphological Classification of Neurons

There are three types of neurons:

1. **Unipolar** found in the dorsal root ganglia
2. **Bipolar** found in the retina, olfactory mucosa, internal ear
3. **Multipolar** found in the cerebrum, cerebellum and anterior horn of spinal cord

### Functional Classification of Neurons

1. **Afferent** or sensory neurons
2. **Efferent** or motor neurons
3. **Interneurons** or connector neurons

## SUPPORTING CELLS (NEUROGLIA) OF CNS

Supporting cells of the central nervous system or neuroglia are a group of nervous tissues which are neither capable of excitability nor can conduct an impulse.

### Types of Neuroglia

1. Astrocytes
   a. Protoplasmic astrocytes
   b. Fibrocytic astrocytes
2. Oligodendrocytes
3. Microglia
4. Ependymal cells

## SUPPORTING CELLS OF PERIPHERAL NERVOUS SYSTEM

1. Schwann cells
2. Satellite cells

The major functions of the supporting cells are as follows:

1. Protection
2. Support
3. Nourishment of neurons
4. Insulation
5. Myelination
6. Phagocytosis
7. Formation of blood brain barrier

## PERIPHERAL NERVES

### Spinal Nerves

Spinal nerves are derived from the spinal segments of spinal cord. There are 31 pairs of spinal nerves. The spinal nerves are named according to the regional segment of origin. Therefore, there are:

- 8 pairs of cervical nerves,
- 12 pairs of thoracic nerves,
- 5 pairs of lumbar nerves,
- 5 pairs of sacral nerves and
- one pair of coccygeal nerves.

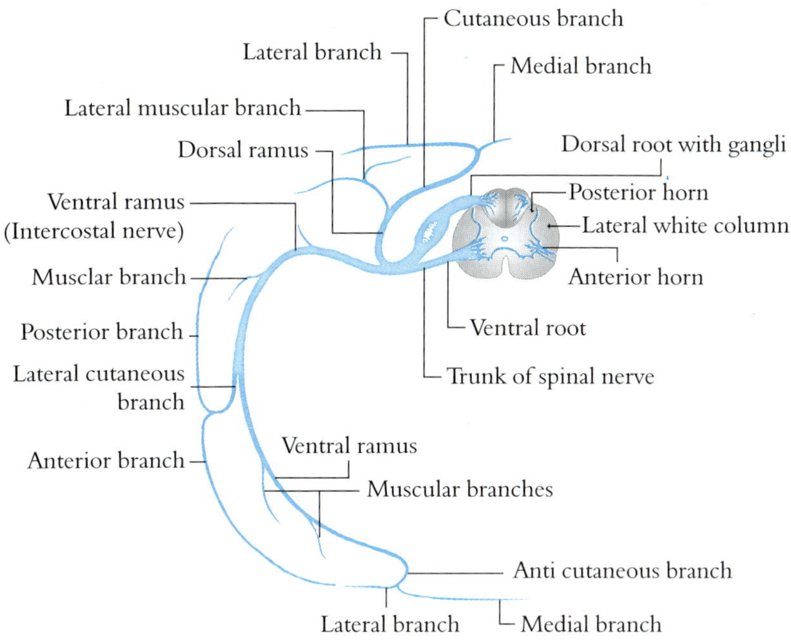


**Fig. 7.1: Typical spinal nerve**

## *Parts and formation of a typical spinal nerve*

Each spinal nerve is formed by the union of:

1. an anterior (ventral) root of the spinal segment and
2. a posterior (dorsal) root of the spinal segment.

The union of both roots takes place within the respective *intervertebral foramen* to form a typical *spinal nerve*. A spinal nerve is very short and is not more than 1mm in length. Each dorsal root just proximal to the union passes through a swelling, *posterior root ganglia*, which contain the cell bodies of sensory neurons. These ganglia also lie within the intervertebral foramina. There are no synapses in these ganglia, they are simply the sites of the cell bodies.

The anterior root contains motor *(efferent)* fibers for skeletal muscles along with autonomic fibers from $T_1$-$L_2$ and $S_2$-$S_4$. The posterior root of every spinal nerve contains sensory *(afferent)* fibers.

Immediately after its formation the spinal nerve divides into:

1. an anterior ramus and
2. a posterior ramus.

It is to be noted that all great nerve plexuses (cervical, brachial, lumbar and sacral) are formed by the anterior rami. Posterior rami of the spinal nerves do not form any plexuses in the body.

## CRANIAL NERVES

These were named cranial nerves due to the presence of their nuclei in the central nervous system. There are 12 pairs of cranial nerves. These are denoted by Roman numerals.

i. Olfactory
ii. Optic
iii. Oculomotor
iv. Trochlear
v. Trigeminal
vi. Abducent
vii. Facial
viii. Vestibulocochlear
ix. Glossopharyngeal
x. Vagus
xi. Accessory
xii. Hypoglossal

## FUNCTIONAL COMPONENTS OF PERIPHERAL NERVES

### Functional Components Common in Both Spinal and Cranial Nerves

1. **General somatic efferents (GSE)** consist of motor fibers that supply the skeletal muscles of limbs and body wall.
2. **General visceral efferents (GVE)** consist of motor fibers of autonomic nervous system which supply the smooth muscles and glands.
3. **General somatic afferents (GSA)** consist of ***exteroceptive*** (sensory fibers of touch, pain, temperature, and pressure)fibers from skin and ***proprioceptive*** (sense of position and movement) fibers from the muscles, joints and tendons.
4. **General visceral afferents (GVA)** consist of ***interoceptive*** (visceroceptive) fibers from viscera and organs. They are concerned

with the sensation of visceral pain, and with the poorly localized sensations of thirst, hunger, respiration and sexual feelings.

### Functional Components Peculiar to Cranial Nerves

1. **Special somatic afferents (SSA)** consist of fibers from ***teleceptors.*** They carry the sensations of vision, smell, hearing and equilibrium.
2. **Special visceral afferents (SVA)** carry the fibers of taste.
3. **Special somatic efferents (SSE)** innervate the muscles of tongue and extraocular muscles.
4. **Special visceral efferents (SVE)** carry impulses from visceral musculature which develops from the pharyngeal arches. They include muscles of facial expression, muscles of mastication, muscles of the pharynx and larynx.

## AUTONOMIC NERVOUS SYSTEM

Autonomic nervous system is concerned with the control and regulation of involuntary activities of the body at the unconscious level e.g. circulation, respiration, perspiration, salivation digestion and sexual drive etc.

The main function of this system is to maintain the internal environment of the body in co-ordination with the endocrine system.

The higher centers controlling and regulating the autonomic nervous system are:

1. Frontal cortex,
2. Hypothalamus and
3. Reticular formation.

There are two main divisions of the autonomic nervous system.

1. Sympathetic division
2. Parasympathetic division

Both the divisions are antagonists of each other. Therefore, both the divisions work in co-ordination to keep equilibrium in the internal environment.

### Sympathetic Chains and Ganglia

These are paired structures extending from first cervical vertebra to the tip of coccyx. It consists of a series of *paravertebral* and *prevertebral* ganglia interconnected with each other. The paravertebral ganglia are called as superior, middle, and inferior cervical and thoracolumbar ganglia ($T_1$-$L_2$), whereas prevertebral ganglia are located around the ventral branches of abdominal aorta and have acquired the names of the respective arteries i.e. coeliac, superior mesenteric and inferior mesenteric ganglia.

## Parasympathetic Outflow and Ganglia

Parasympathetic outflow consists of *craniosacral* outflow. Cranial fibers emerge from edinger westphal nucleus, superior and inferior salivatory nuclei located in the brain stem. The preganglionic fibers reach their respective ganglia via III, VII, and IX cranial nerves. These ganglia are as follows.

1. Ciliary ganglia
2. Pterygopalatine ganglia
3. Submandibular ganglia
4. Otic ganglia

The Nucleus of the X Cranial nerve (vagus) is located in the Medulla oblongata. The preganglionic parasympathetic fibers travel via the vagus nerve to the visceras of the thorax (esophagus lungs and heart) and the abdomen (stomach, small intestine, from colon to the splenic flexure, spleen, liver, galbladder, pancreas and kidneys).

Sacral outflow emerge from $S_3$-$S_4$ spinal segments and constitute the pelvic splanchnic nerves or *nervi erigentes.* These fibers terminate and synapse in the ganglia located on the or within the substance of lower part of colon, uterus, genitals, and sphincters of the bladder and urethra.

The important features of autonomic nervous system are summarized in table 7-1.

**Table 7-1: Comparison of the Sympathetic and Parasympathetic Nervous System**

| S. No | Description | Sympathetic system | Parasympathetic system |
|---|---|---|---|
| 1 | Origin | Thoracolumbar ($T_{12}$- $L_2$) | Craniosacral (brainstem and $S_3$-$S_4$) |
| 2 | Location | Prevertebral and paravertebral and lie close to CNS | Ganglia lie away from CNS nearer to effector organ |

| S. No | Description | Sympathetic system | Parasympathetic system |
|---|---|---|---|
| 3 | Ganglia | Cervical, thoracic, lumbar, and pelvic forming thoracic chain | Ciliary, otic, pterigopalatine, and submandibular having isolate and separate occurrence |
| 4 | Distribution | Through the body | To head, thorax, abdomen and pelvic viscera |
| 5 | Blood vessels | Vasodilatation | Vasoconstriction |
| 6 | Heart | Tachycardia | Bradycardia |
| 7 | GIT motility | Inhibits | Stimulates |
| 8 | GIT secretions | Decrease | Increase |
| 9 | GIT sphincters | Constrict | Relax |
| 10 | Lungs | Bronchodilator | Bronchoconstrictor |
| 11 | Salivary glands | No effect | Secretions increase |
| 12 | Sweat glands | Stimulate (perspiration) | No effect |
| 13 | Lacrimal glands | No effect | Stimulate (lacrimation) |
| 14 | Nasal and palatine glands | No effect | Stimulate (Rhinorrhoea) |
| 15 | Urinary bladder | Bladder relaxes, sphincter constricts | Bladder contracts, sphincter relaxes |
| 16 | Eye | Pupil constricts (Meiosis) | Pupil dilates (Mydriasis) |
| 17 | Sexual organs | Ejaculation | Erection |

# Chapter 8 IMAGING TECHNIQUES

**Exploring** the anatomy of human body by different procedures and techniques remains the most useful and effective tool of diagnostic medicine. The introduction of latest methods of investigations and imaging are now playing a key role in more accurate and perfect diagnosis.

Human body can be explored by two methods.

1. Endoscopy
2. Imaging

## 1. ENDOSCOPY

It is the procedure to directly visualize the internal organs of the body by using fiber optic built-in techniques in the instruments called *endoscopes*. The following procedures are more commonly performed:

### a. Bronchoscopy

Inspection of the interior of tracheobroncheal tree with the help of a *bronchoscope* is called bronchoscopy. It is useful in diagnostic and therapeutic maneuvers e.g. removing a foreign body or taking a specimen for biopsy.

### b. Gastroscopy

Examination of the interior of stomach by the help of a fiber optic endoscope is called as gastroscopy. The instrument used is called a *gastroscope*. It is helpful in diagnosing the gastric erosions, ulcers and tumours.

### c. Laparoscopy

Examination of the peritoneal cavity (interior of abdomen) and performing surgical or diagnostic procedures by means of an instrument called *laparoscope* is called as laparoscopy. It is now becoming one of the most popular techniques in modern surgery. The advantages of this technique are as follows.

a. Small sized incision (just to introduce the laparoscope)
b. Minimal scarring (cosmetic advantage)
c. Mostly done under local anaesthesia, therefore very safe
d. Early rehabilitation

### d. Proctoscopy

It is the procedure to inspect the anal canal and rectum internally by means of a *proctoscope.* However, other instruments like *proctosigmoidoscope* are now in use for inspecting the ascending and sigmoid colon, rectum and anal canal.

### e. Cystoscopy

Visual examination of the urinary tract by means of a *cystoscope* both for diagnostic and treatment purposes is called cystoscopy.

## 2. IMAGING

It is the technique to indirectly visualize the interior of human body. Two main categories of imaging are:

### a. Methods Using the Ionizing Radiations

#### *i. x-rays*

These are electromagnetic rays of short wavelength produced when electrons moving at high velocity impinge on various structures to fluorescence or strongly ionize the tissue. This technique depends on the differential absorption of x-rays by the various tissues of the body. Those structures which absorb most of the x-rays are known as *radiopaque* e.g. teeth and compact bone, whereas substances with least absorption are called as *radiolucent* e.g. air in the lungs, windpipe, stomach, and intestine. The image of the desired structures is obtained on a film coated plate after exposing them to x-rays. Different applications of x-rays are summarized below.

- **Simple radiograph or roentgenogram** consists of conventional plain type of radiographs e.g. x-ray chest, or x-ray knee joint. These radiographs expose only two dimensional images. Therefore, x-rays from different angles are required to assess the diseases.

- **Contrast media radiographs** are required where plain x-rays fail to explore the structures which are invisible otherwise. Different substances are used to enhance the contrast of the structures under observation. Common examples are:
  - Barium sulphate used as *barium meals* or *barium enema* to explore the GIT
  - Organic iodide used in IVP (intravenous pyelography) to find out any pathology in the urinary tract
- **CT scan** or computerized tomography is the method of obtaining cross sectional images of the body structures in the axial planes by using the x-rays.

### *ii. γ-rays*

Gamma rays are electromagnetic radiation of short wavelengths consisting of high energy photons. They have great penetrating power. They are emitted from radioactive elements like $T^{99}$ and Thalium etc. Minute quantities of these radioactive elements are introduced into the body and the rays are picked up and photographed by a special γ-camera. These are used for the following:

- Bone scan
- Thyroid scan
- Hida scan (for liver)
- Renal scan
- Mebe and thalium scans (for heart) etc.

## b. Methods Without Exposure to Radiations

### *i. Ultrasonography (USG)*

Ultrasound *(sonar)* are used to produce echoes or electronic pictures representing the reflection of that ultrasound from tissue interfaces. In this technique, high frequency sound waves called *ultrasound* are used to examine the internal structures. The ultrasounds are directed towards the structure to be examined by a probe or transducer. Different structures reflect the sound waves with different intensity. The reflecting waves are picked up by the same transducer which converts them into electrical signals. The signals produce the echoes or images on the computer screen.

It is a very safe method and is free of any radiation hazards. It is, therefore, used as a method of choice in pregnant women to monitor the progress or abnormalities of the developing embryo in the very early months.

### *ii. Magnetic resonance imaging (MRI)*

It is also a cross sectional topography technique. In this method protons ($H^+$) can be made to resonate in a strong magnetic field when subjected to the appropriate radio wavelength. Such resonations are recorded and processed to compute an electronic image. The main advantage of this technique is that images can be taken in axial, coronal and sagittal planes as compared to CT scan which can only produce images in axial plane. It gives better details and information including the biochemical changes occurring in the body along with its exact location than the CT scan. It is, therefore, more useful in soft tissues imaging. Other advantages include its high intrinsic contrast and safety from radiational hazards.

### *iii. Angiography*

It is the exploration of the vascular pattern of a specific region, viscera or a structure after injecting the fluorescence dye in the blood e.g. angiography of the heart and fundus fluorescein angiography (FFA) of retina.

Chapter

# 9 SEQs

1. a. In a tabulated form, classify skeletal muscles with obliquely arranged muscle fibers giving one example of each type from upper and lower limbs.
   b. What is the range of mobility and force of pull in these muscles?

2. a. Define a spinal nerve and name various spinal nerves existing in human body with their numbers.
   b. Write the pattern of emergence of various spinal nerves from vertebral column.

3. a. Write the anatomical features of "hinge joint".
   b. Write any example of hinge joints present in the limbs and name the movement permitted at the quoted two joints with their common axis of movement.

4. a. What is meant by 'anatomical position' of human body?
   b. Briefly mention four fundamental planes used to study human body.

5. a. In a tabulated form, classify synovial joints according to the arrangement of articular surfaces and quote one example of each from the limbs.
   b. What is *Hilton's law* of nerve supply of joints?

6. a. Define spinal nerves and mention their number in humans.
   b. Write formation of a typical spinal nerve and draw diagram.

7. a. Define the terms Coronal plane, Plain joint, Bicipital muscle, Mechanoreceptors and Apocrine glands.

8. Define complex joint. Mention THREE examples from upper limb. Explain the movements of uniaxial complex joint of upper limb which has pivot structural appearance. Why are screws, nuts, and bolts tightened with the right hand by everyone (irrespective of handedness)?

9. Define pennate muscles; mention their functional significance. Classify them; mention ONE example of each type from lower limb.

10. Write short note on SESAMOID bones. Give one example each from upper limb and lower limb.

11. Classify synovial joints. Give one example of each to illustrate your answer.

12. a. Define and classify FIBROUS JOINTS.
    b. Name at least three types of SUTURES with one example of each.

13. What is the arterial supply of a LONG BONE? Write its venous drainage.

# SECTION 2

# UPPER LIMB

## CONTENTS


| | | |
|---|---|---|
| 10 | Pectoral girdle | 57 |
| 11 | Shoulder | 71 |
| 12 | Axilla and breast | 81 |
| 13 | The arm | 99 |
| 14 | The forearm | 111 |
| 15 | The wrist and hand | 127 |
| 16 | Miscellaneous | 139 |
| 17 | SEQs | 147 |

Chapter

# 10 PECTORAL GIRDLE

**Pectoral** girdle or shoulder girdle is defined as an articulation between the bones of upper limb i.e. scapula and clavicle with the axial skeleton i.e. sternum. The resultant joint formed is *sternoclavicular joint* whereas the appendicular bones unite at *acromioclavicular joint*. The remaining attachment is muscular which accounts for the large range of mobility of the shoulder girdle.

## MUSCLE ATTACHMENTS BETWEEN SHOULDER GIRDLE AND TRUNK

### 1. Providing Direct Attachment

#### *a. Pectoralis minor*

***Origin***

3-4-5$^{th}$ ribs

***Insertion***

Coracoid process

***Nerve supply***

Medial and lateral pectoral nerves (C6, C7, C8)

***Actions***

i. Protraction of scapula
ii. Depresses shoulder (by medial rotation of scapula)
iii. Assists gravity in restoring the normal position of scapula after full abduction

*Significance:* It is an important landmark, being the guide to the axillary artery and the cords of the brachial plexus.

### b. Subclavius

**Origin**

Costal cartilage of first rib

**Insertion**

Subclavian groove at inferior surface of clavicle

**Nerve supply**

Branch of upper trunk of the brachial plexus (C5, C6)

**Action**

Assists in stabilizing the clavicle to sternum in movements of the shoulder girdle

> *Significance:* It prevents the damage to subclavian vein by the segments of clavicle in case of fracture.

### c. Trapezius

**Origin**

i. Medial 1/3 of superior nuchal line
ii. Ligamentum nuchae
iii. Spine of C7 and all 12 thoracic vertebral spines

**Insertion**

i. Upper fibers—lateral 1/3 of clavicle
ii. Middle fibers—medial border of acromion and crest of scapular spine
iii. Lower fibers—medial end of spine of scapula

**Nerve supply**

i. Spinal part of accessory nerve (C1, C2, C3, C4, C5)
ii. Branches from cervical roots (C3, C4, C5)

**Actions**

i. All the fibers retract the scapula.
ii. Upper and lower fibers rotate the scapula and tilt the glenoid cavity upwards to facilitate the overhead abduction of the arm.

iii. Upper fibers elevate the whole shoulder (shrugging of shoulders).

iv. Acting unilaterally: lateral flexion of neck

v. Acting bilaterally: extend the neck

*Significance:* When carrying something heavy, this muscle prevents the depression of shoulder.

### d. Rhomboid major

#### Origin

Spines of T2- T5

#### Insertion

Medial border of scapula (entire length)

#### Nerve supply

Dorsal scapular nerve (C5)

#### Actions

i. Medial rotation of scapula
ii. Elevation of scapula
iii. Retraction of scapula

### e. Rhomboid minor

#### Origin

Spines of C7 and T1

#### Insertion

Root of scapular spine at medial border

#### Nerve supply

Dorsal scapular nerve (C5)

#### Actions

i. Elevation of scapula
ii. Retraction of scapula

### *f. Levator scapulae*

**Origin**

Transverse process of C1, C2, C3, C4

**Insertion**

Medial border of scapula from superior angle to spine

**Nerve supply**

i. Cervical plexus (C3, C4)
ii. Dorsal scapular nerve (C5)

**Actions**

i. Elevation of scapula
ii. Lateral rotation of the neck

### *g. Serratus anterior*

**Origin**

Upper eight ribs

**Insertion**

Medial border of costal surface of scapula

**Nerve supply**

Long thoracic nerve (C5, C6, C7)

**Actions**

i. Protraction of scapula
ii. Lateral rotation of scapula (to assist abduction of arm beyond 90°)

> *Significance:* It is a very strong muscle of *punching and pushing*. It is also called as the *boxer's muscle*.

## 2. Providing Indirect Attachment

### *a. Pectoralis major*

**Origin**

i. Clavicular head—medial 1/2 of clavicle

ii. Sternocostal head
    - Lateral ½ of manubrium and body of sternum
    - Upper six costal cartilages

### Insertion

i. Lateral lip of the intertubercular sulcus
ii. Lowest fibers blend with the capsule of shoulder joint

### Nerve supply

i. Lateral pectoral nerve (C5-6-7)
ii. Medial pectoral nerve (C8-T1)

### Actions

i. Flexion—clavicular head
ii. Adduction of arm (most powerful)—sternocostal head
iii. Medial rotation of arm—both heads
iv. Accessory muscle of inspiration

> *Significance:* It is the only muscle of the upper limb which is supplied by all five segments of brachial plexus (C5-T1).

## b. Latissimus dorsi

### Origin

i. Spines of the lower six thoracic vertebrae
ii. Lumbar fascia
iii. Outer lip of iliac crest

### Insertion

Floor of the intertubercular sulcus

### Nerve supply

Thoracodorsal nerve (C6, C7, C8)

### Actions

i. Extension of shoulder joint

ii. Medial rotation of arm
iii. Adduction of arm

*Significance:*

1. It is essentially the *climbing muscle*.
2. It is the only muscle of the upper limb to have a pelvic attachment (via lumbar fascia).
3. The myocutaneous flap of this muscle is often used by the surgeons in reconstructive surgery of breast.

## CLAVIPECTORAL FASCIA

It is a strong fascial sheet extending between the clavicle and pectoralis minor. The fused layers of the fascia below the subclavius extend between the coracoids process and first costochondral junction as a strong membrane called as *costocoracoid ligament*.

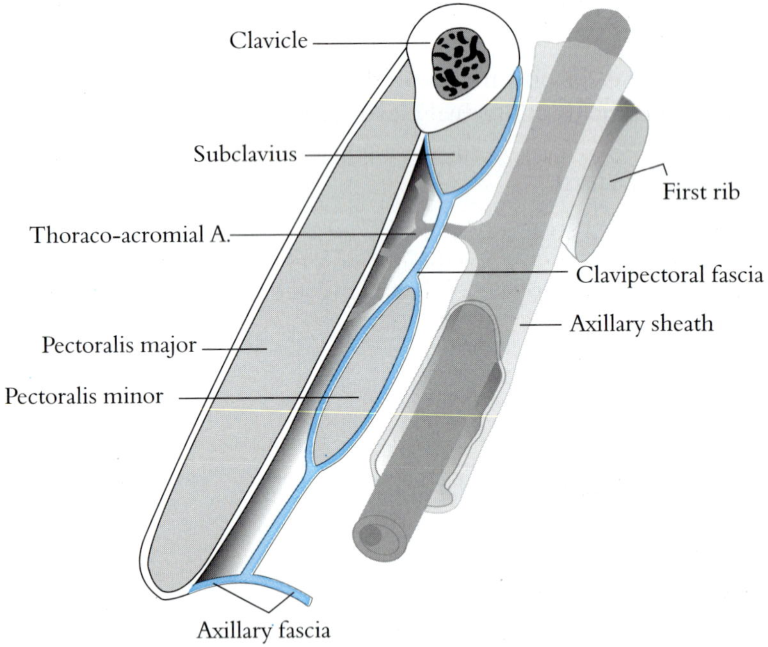


**Fig. 10.1: Clavipectoral fascia**

### Attachments

- **Laterally**—coracoid process
- **Medially**—external intercostal membrane of upper two spaces
- **Superiorly**—splits into two layers to enclose subclavius and then attaches to the under surface of the clavicle
- **Inferiorly**—splits to enclose pectoralis minor muscle and then extend downwards as the *suspensory ligament of the axilla* which blends with the axillary fascia over the axillary floor

### Muscles Invested by the Fascia

1. Subclavius
2. Pectoralis minor

### Structures Piercing Through the Fascia

*Passing inwards:*

1. Cephalic vein
2. Lymphatics from infraclavicular nodes to the apical group of axilla

*Passing outwards:*

1. Lateral pectoral nerve
2. Thoracoacromial artery or its branches

*Significance:* It maintains the hollow of the axilla (arm pit) by keeping the axillary fascia tense through the suspensory ligament of the axilla.

## MOVEMENTS OF THE SCAPULA

### Protraction

1. Serratus anterior
2. Pectoralis major
3. Pectoralis minor

### Retraction

1. Trapezius—middle fibers
2. Rhomboid major
3. Rhomboid minor

### Elevation

1. Levator scapulae
2. Trapezius—upper fibers

### Depression

1. Pectoralis minor and major
2. Trapezius—lower fibers
3. Latissimus dorsi

### Lateral Rotation

1. Trapezius—upper fibers
2. Serratus anterior

### Medial Rotation

1. Levator scapulae
2. Rhomboids
3. Latissimus dorsi
4. Gravity

*Significance:* Protraction is the movement used in punching and pushing. Rotator movements are used in overhead abduction and adduction of the arm.

## TRIANGLE OF AUSCULTATION

It is a small gap between the muscles of the back near the inferior angle of the scapula. It lies and becomes subcutaneous to the sixth intercostals space when both the arms flex anteriorly in a crossing manner on the chest.

### *Boundaries*

**Superior:** Trapezius

**Inferior:** Latissimus dorsi

**Lateral:** Scapula (medial border)

**Floor:** Rhomboid major

*Significance:* This small muscular gap is the best and usual place to listen (or auscultate) the lung sounds posteriorly by the stethoscope.

## INTERMUSCULAR SPACES

### 1. Quadrangular Space

#### *Boundaries*

**Superior:** Subscapularis, teres minor

**Inferior:** Teres major

**Medial:** Long head of triceps

**Lateral:** Surgical neck of humerus

#### *Contents*

1. Axillary nerve
2. Posterior circumflex humeral artery and vein

### 2. Upper Triangular Space

#### *Boundaries*

**Superior:** Teres minor

**Inferior:** Teres major

**Lateral:** Long head of triceps

#### *Contents*

Circumflex scapular artery

### 3. Lower Triangular Space

#### *Boundaries*

**Superior:** Teres major

**Medial:** Long head of triceps

**Lateral:** Medial border of humerus

#### *Contents*

1. Radial nerve
2. Profunda brachial artery and vein

## STERNOCLAVICULAR JOINT

### Type

Synovial joint (saddle type) of atypical variety, because the articulating surfaces of the joint are covered by fibrocartilage instead of hyaline cartilage. Functionally, it behaves like a ball and socket joint.

### Articulating Bones

1. Medial end of clavicle
2. Superolateral part of manubrium sterni
3. First costal cartilage

**Fulcrum of movements** of sternoclavicular joint is the *costoclavicular ligament*. Thus when the lateral end of the clavicle moves upwards, the medial end moves downwards.

**Joint cavity:** Joint is separated into two cavities by intervening fibrocartilage.

**Joint capsule:** It is a sleeve like covering which invests the joint externally. It also thickens at two places to form anterior and posterior sternoclavicular ligaments.

**Articular disc** is attached to the capsule, clavicle, and first costal cartilage. It divides the joint cavity into two separate synovial cavities. Its important functions are the following:

1. Prevention of upward dislocation
2. Acting as a shock absorber of compression forces applied from upper limb

### Ligaments

1. Costoclavicular ligament: It has two laminae—anterior and posterior and is the major stabilizing factor of this joint. It takes all strain off the joint. It transmits the stress from the clavicle to first costal cartilage.
2. Interclavicular ligament
3. Anterior sternoclavicular ligament
4. Posterior sternoclavicular ligament

### *Nerve supply*

Supraclavicular nerves

### *Blood supply*

1. Suprascapular artery
2. Internal thoracic artery

### Movements

1. Elevation *(shrugging of the shoulder)*
2. Depression
3. Forward and backward *(squaring of the shoulders)*
4. Rotatory movements are passive and occur during the overhead abduction of arm when scapula rotates.

> *Significance:* Sternoclavicular is the only joint which connects the upper limb with the axial skeleton.

## SCAPULAR ANASTOMOSIS

The arteries participating in the arterial anastomosis around the scapula are summarized below in Table 10-1.

**Table 10-1: Summary of Scapular Anastomosis**

| S.No | Artery | Origin | Supply |
|---|---|---|---|
| 1 | Dorsal scapular artery | Transverse cervical artery, a branch of thyrocervical trunk | Medial border of scapula as far as inferior angle |
| 2 | Suprascapular artery | Thyrocervical trunk, a branch of first part of subclavian artery | Supraspinous and infraspinous fossa |
| 3 | Subscapular artery | Third part of axillary artery | Subscapular fossa |

| | | | |
|---|---|---|---|
| 4 | Circumflex scapular artery | Subscapular artery | Infraspinous fossa |
| 5 | Thoracodorsal artery | Subscapular artery | Lower half of medial border of scapula |

*Significance:* The scapular anastomosis connects the first part of subclavian artery with the third part of axillary artery. It provides an alternate channel of (collateral) circulation when either of these arteries is blocked.

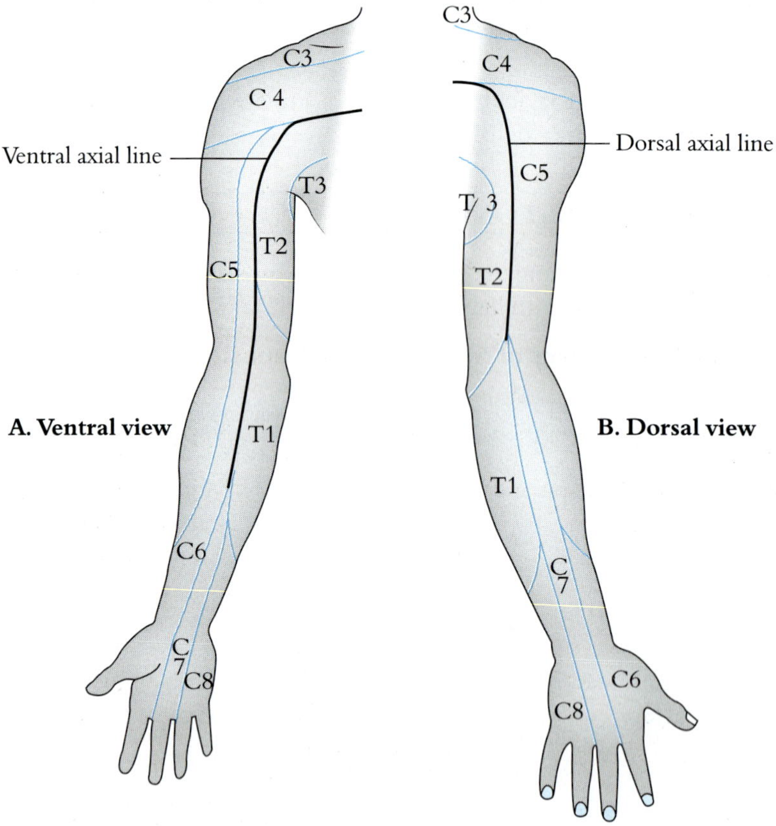


**Fig. 10.2: Dermatomes of the upper limb**

## CUTANEOUS NERVES OF THE UPPER LIMB

**Table 10-2: The Cutaneous Nerves of the Upper Limb**

| S.No | Name | Origin | Distribution |
|---|---|---|---|
| 1 | Supraclavicular nerves | Cervical plexus | Skin over the clavicle and upper part of deltoid and lateral part of pectoralis major |
| 2 | Intercostobrachial nerve | T1-T2 | Skin of axilla and upper medial aspect of arm |
| 3 | Upper lateral cutaneous nerve of the arm | Axillary nerve | Skin over lower lateral part of deltoid |
| 4 | Lower lateral cutaneous nerve of the arm | Radial nerve | Skin over lower lateral aspect of the arm |
| 5 | Medial cutaneous nerve of arm | Medial cord of brachial plexus | Skin over lower medial aspect of the arm |
| 6 | Posterior cutaneous nerve of the arm | Radial nerve | Skin over posterior aspect of the arm |
| 7 | Lateral cutaneous nerve of the forearm | Musculo-cutaneous nerve | Skin over anterolateral part of forearm to wrist |
| 8 | Medial cutaneous nerve of the forearm | Medial cord of brachial plexus | Skin of anteromedial aspect of forearm to wrist |
| 9 | Posterior cutaneous nerve of forearm | Radial nerve | Skin over posterior aspect of forearm to wrist |
| 10 | Superficial branch of radial nerve | Radial nerve | Skin over the dorsum of thumb, index, middle and half of ring finger |

| S.No | Name | Origin | Distribution |
|---|---|---|---|
| 11 | Posterior cutaneous branch of ulnar nerve | Ulnar nerve | Skin over the dorsum of little and half of ring finger |
| 12 | Palmar cutaneous branches of ulnar nerve | Ulnar nerve | Skin over the palm of little and half of ring finger |
| 13 | Palmar cutaneous branches of median nerve | Median nerve | Skin over the palm of thumb, index, middle and half of ring finger |

## CLINICAL AND APPLIED INTEGRATION

### Winging of Scapula

It is a condition which occurs due to the paralysis of the serratus anterior muscle. Long thoracic nerve, a branch of C5, C6 and C7 roots of brachial plexus, damage is the cause. The muscle keeps the medial (vertebral) border of the scapula in firm apposition with the chest. In paralysis of serratus anterior medial border of the scapula becomes prominently raised off the posterior chest wall called as *winging of scapula*.

Chapter

# 11 SHOULDER

**A** group of six muscles surrounding the shoulder converge from the scapula onto the humerus. They strengthen and stabilize the shoulder joint. All the muscles lie under cover of deltoid and trapezius.

## MUSCLES OF THE SHOULDER

### 1. Deltoid

***Origin***

a. *Anterior fibers*—lateral 1/3 of clavicle
b. *Middle fibers*—lateral border of acromion
c. *Posterior fibers*—spine of scapula (inferior lip of the crest)

***Insertion***

Deltoid tuberosity of humerus

***Nerve supply***

Axillary nerve (C5, C6)

***Actions***

a. *Anterior fibers*—flexion and medial rotation of the arm
b. *Middle fibers*—abduction of the arm from 15° through 90°
c. *Posterior fibers*—extension and lateral rotation of the arm

> *Significance:* It is the commonest site for intramuscular injection at the lateral bulge, not more than 4cm below the lower border of acromion to avoid damage to axillary nerve.

### 2. Subscapularis

***Origin***

Subscapular fossa

***Insertion***

Lesser tubercle of humerus

***Nerve supply***

Upper and lower subscapular nerves (C5, C6)

***Actions***

a. Medial rotation of humerus
b. Stabilizaion of shoulder joint

## 3. Supraspinatus

***Origin***

Supraspinatus fossa

***Insertion***

Upper facet of greater tubercle

***Nerve supply***

Suprascapular nerve (C5, C6)

***Actions***

a. Initiates abduction of the arm through 0-15°
b. Stabilization of shoulder joint

## 4. Infraspinatus

***Origin***

Infraspinous fossa

***Insertion***

Central facet of greater tubercle of humerus

***Nerve supply***

Suprascapular nerve (C5, C6)

### *Actions*

a. Lateral rotation of humerus
b. Stabilization of shoulder joint

## 5. Teres Major

### *Origin*

Inferior angle of scapula

### *Insertion*

Medial lip of intertubercular sulcus of humerus

### *Nerve supply*

Lower subscapular nerve (C5, C6)

### *Actions*

a. Adduction of arm
b. Medial rotation of arm
c. Steadying the upper end of humerus in movements

> *Significance:* Teres major may be transplanted posteriorly to provide lateral rotation in case of paralysis of infraspinatus and teres minor.

## 6. Teres Minor

### *Origin*

Lateral border of scapula

### *Insertion*

Lowest facet of greater tubercle of humerus

### *Nerve supply*

Axillary nerve (C5, C6)

### *Actions*

a. Lateral rotation of arm
b. Stabilization of shoulder joint

## SHOULDER JOINT

### Type

It is a synovial joint of ball and socket variety. It is also called as *glenohumeral joint*. This joint is inherently unstable due to the following.

1. Disproportionate size (4:1 ratio) of the head of humerus and the shallow glenoid cavity
2. Lax articular capsule
3. Inadequate inferior support
4. Wide range of movements

### Articulating Bones

1. Head of the humerus
2. Glenoid cavity of scapula
3. Coracoid process
4. Lateral end of the clavicle

### Articular Capsule

It is a thin capsule covered by overlying muscles. It is strengthened by the partly fused tendons of muscles which surround the joint. The capsule consists of:

1. Outer *fibrous membrane and*
2. Inner *synovial membrane.*

**Fibrous membrane** of the capsule is a thin but relatively strong, tubular covering. It is attached to the:

1. Margins of glenoid cavity,
2. Anatomical neck of humerus except inferiorly,
3. Surgical neck inferiorly and
4. Anteriorly bridging the intertubercular sulcus.

There are gaps in the anterior and posterior part of the fibrous capsule which allows communication between the synovial membrane and the subscapularis and infraspinatus bursa anteriorly and posteriorly respectively.

**Synovial membrane** is attached between the glenoid labrum and articular margins of the head of humerus. It lines the capsule internally. It invests the long head of biceps like a tubular sleeve to facilitate gliding of the tendon of this muscle.

## Bursae

1. Subscapular bursa
2. Infraspinatus bursa
3. Subacromial bursa (largest of all)

Subacromial (subdeltoid) bursa lies below the coracoacromial arch and deltoid. It helps in abduction of the arm and protects the friction of supraspinatus tendon with the acromion during the overhead abduction of greater tuberosity of humerus.

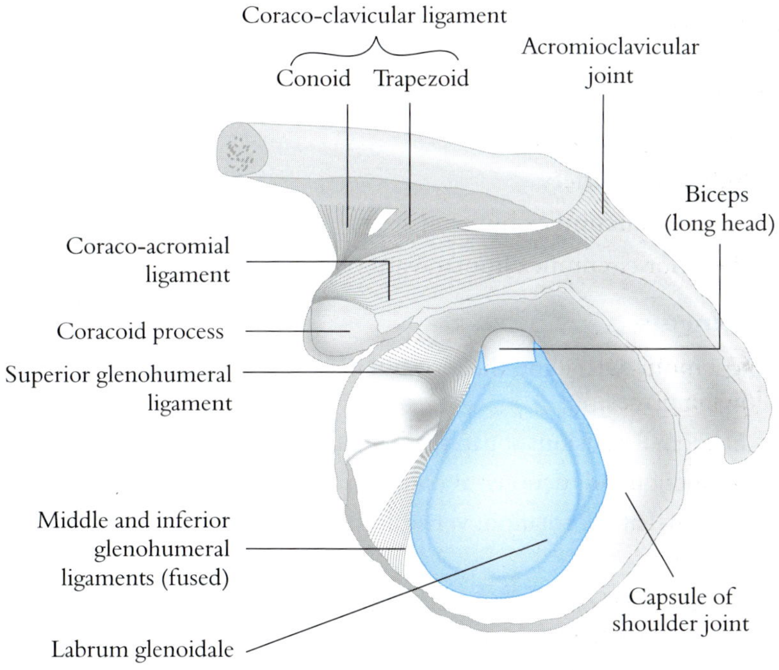


**Fig. 11.1: Capsule and ligaments of the shoulder joint**

## Ligaments

These are four band-like thickenings in the fibrous part of the capsule.

These provide reinforcement to the capsule during movements of the shoulder joint.

1. Coracohumeral ligament
2. Glenohumeral ligaments are a group of three bands:
   a. Superior band
   b. Middle band
   c. Inferior band
3. Coracoacromial ligament
4. Transverse humeral ligament

## Nerve Supply of Shoulder Joint

1. Axillary nerve
2. Musculocutaneous nerve
3. Suprascapular nerve

## Blood Supply of Shoulder Joint

1. Suprascapular artery
2. Subscapular artery
3. Anterior circumflex humeral artery
4. Posterior circumflex humeral artery

## Movements

Being a multi-axial joint, the movements at shoulder joint occur in the following planes.

1. Flexion-Extension: at paramedian plane
2. Abduction-Adductions: at coronal plane
3. Medial-Lateral rotation: vertical axis through humerus shaft

   *Flexion:*

   a. Pectoralis major—clavicular head
   b. Deltoid—anterior fibers
   c. Coracobrachialis
   d. Short head of biceps brachii

   *Extension:*

   a. Latissimus dorsi
   b. Teres major

c. Deltoid—posterior fibers
d. Pectoralis major—sternocostal fibers

*Abduction:*

a. Supraspinatus 0-15° (initiates abduction)
b. Deltoid—middle fibers 15-90° (main abductor)
c. Lateral rotators facilitate 90°-120° (by rotating the arm laterally)
d. Trapezius 120°-180° (by rotating the scapula)
e. Serratus anterior 120°-180° (by rotating the scapula)

> For every 3° abduction of the arm, 2° abduction occurs in the shoulder and 1° occurs by rotation of the scapula.

*Adduction:*

a. Pectoralis major
b. Latissimus dorsi
c. Teres major
d. Gravity

*Medial rotation:*

a. Subscapularis
b. Teres major

*Lateral rotation:*

a. Infraspinatus
b. Teres minor

*Circumduction:*

It is a combination of movements in orderly sequence of flexion, abduction, extension and adduction or in reverse order.

## Factors Stabilizing the Shoulder Joint

1. **Bony factors**: Coracoacromial arch superiorly
2. **Ligaments**
   a. Glenohumeral ligament
   b. Coracohumeral ligament
   c. Coracoacromial ligament

3. **Muscles:** Partial fusion of the tendons of (rotator cuff) muscles with the joint capsule
   a. Supraspinatus
   b. Infraspinatus
   c. Subscapularis
   d. Teres minor
4. **Glenoid labrum:** Deepening of the glenoid cavity by the labrum
5. **Splinting effect:** Tendons of the long heads of :
   a. Biceps brachii supporting from above and
   b. Triceps supporting from above and below.

## Rotator Cuff

It is a group of four small scapular muscles (abbreviated as SITS) which are the prime rotators of the humerus, except the supraspinatus.

These surround the shoulder like a cuff except inferiorly, and fuse with the capsule of shoulder joint.

They are sometimes also referred to as *intrinsic muscles* of *the shoulder.* The tone of these muscles assists in holding the head of the humerus during the movements at the shoulder joint. The muscles included are summarized in Table 11-1.

**Table 11-1: Summary of Rotator Cuff (SITS) Muscles**

| S. No | Muscle | Nerve supply | Action |
|---|---|---|---|
| 1 | Supraspinatus | Suprascapular nerve | Not a rotator (Abductor) |
| 2 | Infraspinatus | Suprascapular nerve | Lateral rotator of arm |
| 3 | Teres minor | Axillary nerve | Lateral rotator of arm |
| 4 | Subscapularis | Upper and lower subscapular nerves | Medial rotator of arm |

*Significance:* The rotator cuff muscle tendons partially blend with the fibrous capsule of the shoulder joint to form a musculotendinous cuff. This cuff prevents the dislocation of shoulder joint and is one of the major factors which provides stability to this joint. However, this cuff is deficient inferiorly and the joint is relatively weak here.

## CLINICAL AND APPLIED INTEGRATION

### Site of Intramuscular Injection

Deltoid is the commonest muscle used for intramuscular injection. The site for intramuscular injection into deltoid is on the lateral bulge of the shoulder as far as 4cm below the acromion. Beyond it there is a danger of damage to the anterior branch of axillary nerve.

### Frozen Shoulder

It is a condition characterized by pain and restriction of movements of the arm. Overhead abduction is especially affected due to the inflammation of supraspinatus tendon. Rotator cuff tendinitis and adhesive capsulitis (of shoulder joint) are two important causes. The condition may take 12-18 months before it resolves, sometimes without any treatment.

### Dislocation of the Shoulder Joint

Shoulder joint is the most unstable and frequently dislocated joint in the body. A sudden force applied along the axis of the humerus usually displaces the head inferiorly when it is abducted above the shoulder and laterally rotated. It is mostly dislocated inferiorly because the joint capsule is least supported here. Anterior dislocations are less common whereas posterior dislocations are rare. *Recurrent dislocations* are very common once the joint capsule or the labrum is damaged.

*Axillary nerve* is the most vulnerable structure to damage in inferior dislocation of shoulder joint because it lies directly below the joint capsule. Damage to axillary nerve presents as:

1. Loss of abduction beyond $15^{\circ}$
2. Sensory loss over upper half of deltoid
3. Loss of shoulder contour (bulge)

## The Painful ARC Syndrome

It is a condition characterized by the presence of a spasm and pain in an arc of 50°-130° during overhead abduction of the arm. It is caused by the inflammation of the supraspinatus tendon associated with impingement of the tendon on the coracoacromial bursa. In advance cases supraspinatus tendon may rupture. Severe pain limits the movements of the shoulder joint.

Chapter

# 12 AXILLA AND BREAST

**Axilla** is a pyramidal space between the upper arm and the lateral chest wall. The lower limit of the axilla (i.e. floor) lies at the level of fourth rib. It acts as a passage for the structures passing from the neck to the upper limb and side wall of the thorax.

## AXILLA

### *Boundaries*

#### *Anterior wall*

It extends from the clavicle to anterior axillary fold. It consists of:

1. Clavipectoral fascia,
2. Pectoralis major,
3. Pectoralis minor and
4. Subclavius.

#### *Posterior wall*

It lies between the lateral part of subscapular fossa and the posterior axillary fold. It consists of:

1. Subscapularis and
2. Teres major.

#### *Medial wall*

It is the convex lateral wall of the thorax. It spans on the

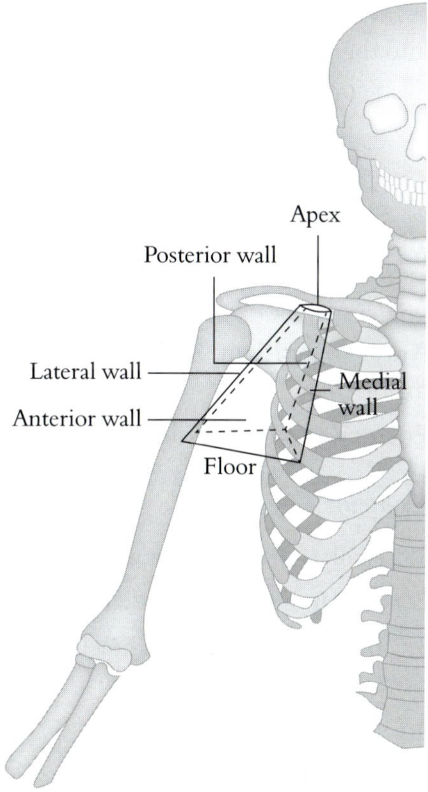


**Fig. 12.1: Walls (boundaries) of the axilla**

first five ribs and corresponding intercostals spaces. It is formed by:

1. Serratus anterior (upper part)

### *Lateral wall*

It is constituted by the upper part of the humerus. The muscles covering it are:

1. Short head of biceps brachii and
2. Coracobrachialis.

### *Apex*

It is a triangular passage through which axilla communicates with the superior thoracic aperture and root of the neck. This passage is called *cervicoaxillary canal.* Axillary neurovascular bundle descends through it into the axilla. The apex is bound by the:

1. Clavicle,
2. First rib and
3. Upper border of scapula.

### *Floor*

Axillary fascia

**Anterior axillary fold** is formed by the lower border of pectoralis major.

**Posterior axillary fold** is formed by the tendon of latissimus dorsi.

### *Contents*

1. Axillary artery and branches
2. Axillary vein and tributaries
3. Infraclavicular part of brachial plexus (i.e., medial, lateral, posterior cords and their branches)
4. Long thoracic nerve
5. Intercostobrachial nerve
6. Axillary lymph nodes
7. Loose adipose tissues

## AXILLARY ARTERY

It is the main source of arterial supply to the upper limb. Pectoralis minor acts as a landmark to trace it. It is divided into three parts for the purpose of description with reference to pectoralis minor.

- First part lies above the muscle.
- Second part lies behind the muscle.
- Third part lies below the muscle.

### *Origin*

It is the continuation of the third part of the *subclavian artery*. It commences at the outer border of the first rib. It enters the axilla behind the midpoint of clavicle.

### *Termination*

It continues as *brachial artery* behind the lower border of teres major.

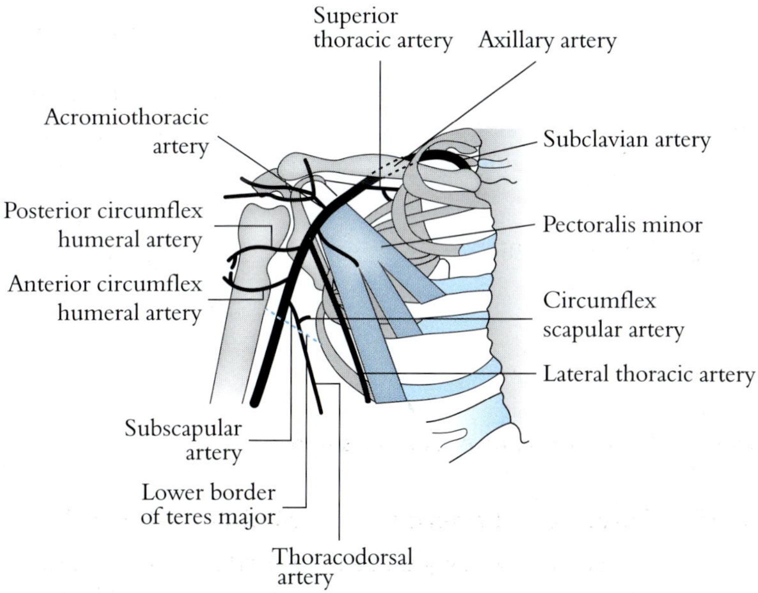


**Fig. 12.2: Course, relations and branches of axillary artery**

**Table 12-1: Branches and Supply of the Axillary Artery**

| Part | Branches | Sub-branches | Supply |
|---|---|---|---|
| 1st part | 1. Superior thoracic artery | | Both pectoral muscles |
| 2nd part | 2. Thoracoacromial artery | a. Clavicular | Clavicle |
| | | b. Deltoid | Deltoid-anterior part |
| | | c. Acromial | Acromion |
| | | d. Pectoral | Pectoral muscles |
| | 3. Lateral thoracic artery | | • Pectoral muscles<br>• Serratus anterior<br>• Lateral half of breast |
| 3rd part | 4. Subscapular artery | a. Circumflex scapular | Scapular muscles |
| | | b. Thoracodorsal | • Latissimus dorsi<br>• Serratus anterior |
| | 5. Ant. Circumflex humeral | | • Shoulder joint<br>• Biceps brachii<br>• Coracobrachialis |
| | 6. Post. Circumflex humeral | | • Shoulder joint<br>• Deltoid<br>• Triceps |

## Relations

**Table 12-2: Relations of Axillary Artery**

| Region | Anterior | Posterior | Medial | Lateral |
|---|---|---|---|---|
| 1st part | • Pectoralis major<br>• Cephalic vein | • Long thoracic nerve | • Axillary vein | • All cords of brachial plexus |

| Region | Anterior | Posterior | Medial | Lateral |
|---|---|---|---|---|
| 2nd part | • Pectoralis minor<br>• Pectoralis major | • Subscapularis<br>• Posterior cord | • Axillary vein<br>• Medial cord | • Lateral cord |
| 3rd part | • Pectoralis major<br>• Medial root of median nerve | • Subscapularis<br>• Latissimus dorsi<br>• Axillary nerve<br>• Radial nerve | • Axillary vein<br>• Ulnar nerve<br>• Medial cutaneous nerve of the arm | • Biceps<br>• Coracobrachialis<br>• Musculocutaneous N<br>• Lat. root of median N |

## AXILLARY VEIN

### *Origin*

It is the continuation of the basilic vein. It commences at the lower border of the teres major.

### *Termination*

It ends at the outer border of the first rib and becomes the subclavian vein.

### *Relations*

It lies medial to axillary artery and partly overlaps it anteriorly.

### *Tributaries*

1. Cephalic vein
2. Venae comitantes of the brachial artery
3. Corresponding branches of axillary artery

### Axillary Sheath

It is the prolongation of the prevertebral part of deep fascia of the neck. It invests the axillary artery and infraclavicular part of the brachial plexus. However, it does not envelop the subclavian or axillary veins so that it can dilate freely in case of increased venous return.

## VEINS OF THE UPPER LIMB

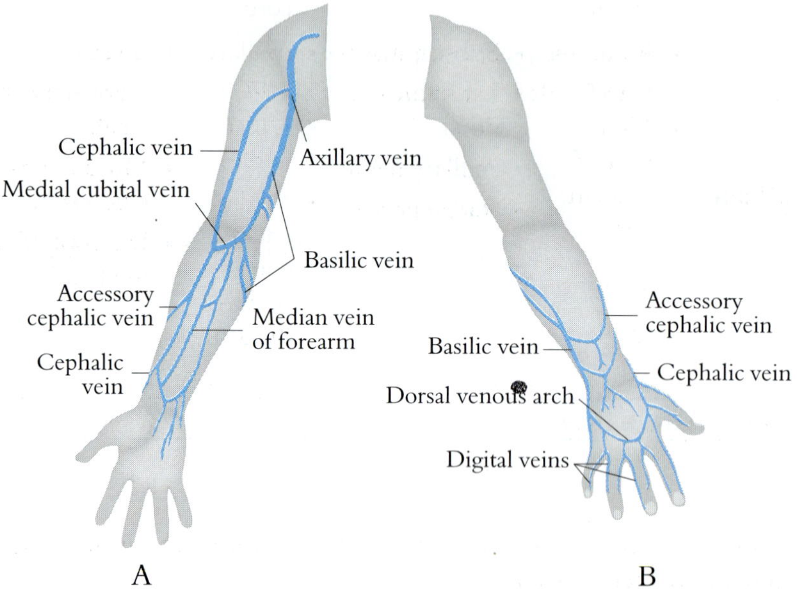


**Fig. 12.3: Veins of the upper limb (A) front (B) back view**

## BRACHIAL PLEXUS

### Formation

The formation of brachial plexus occurs in the following sequence.

### Roots

Ventral (anterior) rami of C5, C6, C7, C8 and T1 of spinal nerves. The five roots lie behind the scalenus anterior muscle.

### Trunks

The roots emerge between the scalenus anterior and scalenus medius to form trunks.

- The upper two roots i.e., C5 and C6 unite to form the *upper trunk*.

- The central root i.e., C7 continues as the *middle trunk*.
- The lower two roots i.e., C7 and C8 unite to form the *lower trunk*.

## Divisions

Each of the three trunks divides into an *anterior* and a *posterior division* behind the clavicle. Hence, three anterior and three posterior divisions are formed.

## Cords

Formation of cords takes place at the outer border of the first rib which then enter the axilla.

- Upper two anterior divisions unite to form the *lateral cord*.
- The anterior division of the lower trunk runs on as *medial cord*.
- All the three posterior divisions unite to form the *posterior cord*.

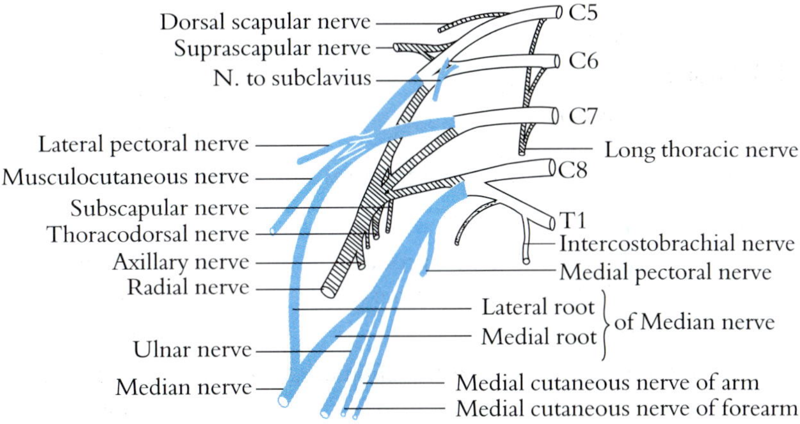


**Fig. 12.4: Formation and branches of brachial plexus**

## Relations in the Axilla

The three cords enter the axilla above the first part of axillary artery. Each lie lateral, medial, and posterior to the second part of the artery respectively according to its title name. The cords give off branches in their prime relations around the third part of axillary artery.

## Branches of the Brachial Plexus

### Table 12-3: Branches and Supply of the Brachial Plexus

| Source | Origin | Branches | Supply |
|---|---|---|---|
| Roots | *C5* | 1. Dorsal scapular nerve | • Rhomboids major and minor<br>• Levator scapulae |
| | *C5, C6, C7* | 2. Long thoracic nerve | • Serratus anterior |
| Trunks | *Upper* | 1. Nerve to subclavius | • Subclavius |
| | | 2. Suprascapular nerve | • Supraspinatus<br>• Infraspinatus<br>• Shoulder joint<br>• Acromioclavicular joints |
| Divisions | *Anterior* | Nil | • Flexor compartment |
| | *Posterior* | Nil | • Extensor compartment |
| Cords | *Lateral cord* | 1. Lateral pectoral nerve | • Pectoralis major and minor |
| | | 2. Lateral root of median nerve | • Joins the medial root to forms median nerve |
| | | 3. Musculocutaneous nerve | • Coracobrachialis, biceps, brachialis |
| | | • Lat. cutaneous N of forearm | • Skin over lateral aspect of forearm |
| | *Medial cord* | 1. Medial pectoral nerve | • Pectoralis minor and major |
| | | 2. Medial root of median nerve | • Forms median nerve with lateral root, continuation of the cord |

| Source | Origin | Branches | Supply |
|---|---|---|---|
| **Cords** (cont.) | *Medial cord* | 3. Medial Cutaneous N of arm | • Skin over front and medial side of arm |
| | | 4. Med. Cutaneous N of forearm | • Skin over lower part of arm and medial side of forearm |
| | | 5. Ulnar nerve | • Supplies small muscles of the hand, largest branch of medial cord |
| | *Posterior cord* | 1. Upper subscapular nerve | • Upper part of subscapularis |
| | | 2. Lower subscapular nerve | • Latissimus dorsi |
| | | 3. Thoracodorsal nerve | • Lower part of subscapularis<br>• Teres major |
| | | 4. Axillary nerve<br>a. anterior branch<br>b. posterior branch<br>c. upper lateral cutaneous N of the arm | • Shoulder joint<br>• Deltoid<br>• Teres minor<br>• Skin over the upper lateral surface of arm |
| | | 5. Radial nerve<br>a. posterior cutaneous N of arm | • Long and medial head of triceps<br>• Skin over the posterior surface of upper arm |

Radial nerve is the largest branch of the whole brachial plexus. It is the nerve of the extensor compartment of the upper limb.

### *Variations of formation*

**Pre-fixed brachial plexus:** The origin of the plexus shifts one segment upwards with the contribution from C4 whereas that of T1 is absent.

**Post-fixed brachial plexus:** The origin of the plexus shifts one segment down with the contribution from T2 whereas that of C4 is absent.

## CLINICAL AND APPLIED INTEGRATION

### Accessory Phrenic Nerve

C5 is a branch frequently given off by the nerve to subclavius. It provides an alternate pathway for some C5 fibers to reach the diaphragm.

## LESIONS OF BRACHIAL PLEXUS

### Nerve of Bell and Winging of the Scapula

This is the name given to long thoracic nerve which originates from C5, C6 and C8 roots of the brachial plexus and supplies the serratus anterior muscle. It is called so because serratus anterior helps for ringing the bell (in the church). It can be injured by blows or pressure on the posterior triangle of the neck. It presents with the **winging of scapula**.

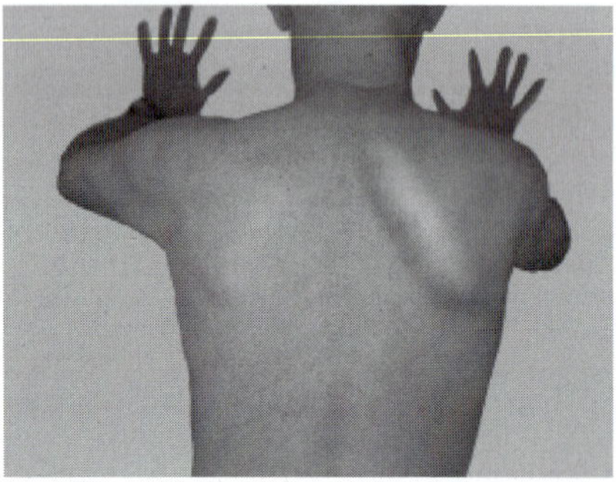

Fig. 12.5: Winging of the scapula

### ERB'S (Duchenne) Paralysis

It is the lesion of the *upper trunk* (C5, C6) of brachial plexus at ERB's point. It is characterized by the typical posture of *waiter's tip or policeman's* tip. The limb of the affected side is medially rotated and hangs by the side. This deformity presents with the follows:

1. Loss of abduction of arm

2. Loss of lateral rotation
3. The arm medially rotated
4. Pronation of the affected forearm
5. Sensory loss over the lower part of deltoid

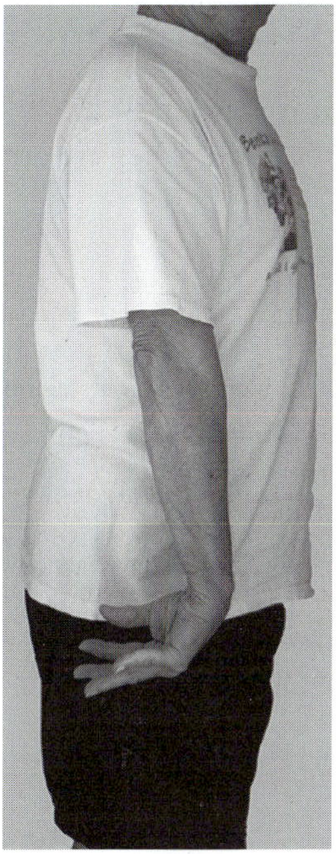

**Fig. 12.6: ERB'S paralysis showing typical condition**

## Klumpke's Paralysis

This disability is caused by injury to the *lower trunk* (C8, T1) of the brachial plexus. The common causes are excessive pull of upper limb of a baby during delivery. Another common cause is over-abduction of the arm during a sudden fall to catch something. The flexors of the ulnar side of wrist and fingers along with the intrinsic muscles of hand are affected. This condition presents with:

1. The ulnar claw hand,
2. Loss of cutaneous sensation over the ulnar border of forearm and
3. Horner's syndrome, a condition resulting by the damage of sympathetic fibers as the sympathetic fibers to the head and neck leave through T1.

## Crutch Paralysis and Saturday Night Paralysis

The compression paralysis of one or both of the upper limbs due to pressure of crutch in the axilla is known as *crutch paralysis*. The axillary nerve is affected by constant compression in this condition. A similar condition called *Saturday night paralysis* is usually seen in Western society. At the weekends people relax and some of them become drunken. Under the influence of alcohol people go into deep sleep in the chair with one arm hanging over the back of chair. As a result the contents of the axilla (axilary nerve) are compressed leading to the paralysis of the hanging limb.

## AXILLARY LYMPH NODES

It is a group of 20-30 lymph nodes scattered in the fibrofatty layer of the axilla. They are arranged in the following groups:

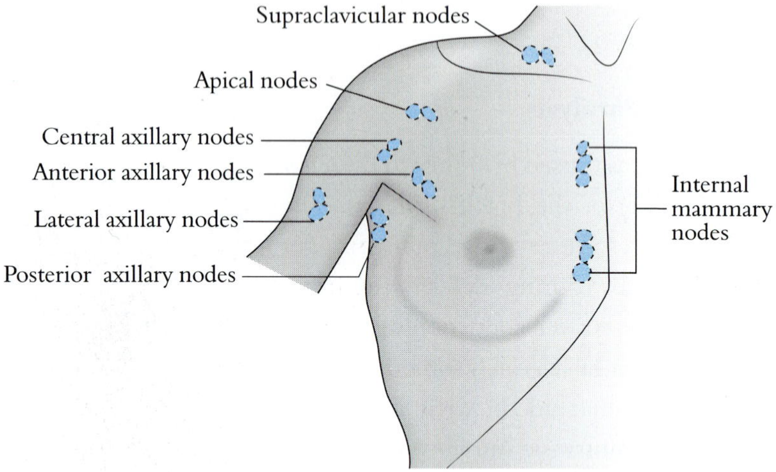


**Fig. 12.7: Lymph nodes of the pectoral region and the axilla**

### 3. Anterior (Pectoral) Group

*Location:*

It lies along the medial wall of axilla with lateral thoracic artery, at the lower border of pectoralis minor.

*Receives lymph from:*

Upper half of trunk

Major part of breast

### 4. Posterior (Subscapular) Group

*Location:*

It is located in the medial wall of axilla in the posterior part along the subscapular artery.

*Receives lymph from:*

Upper half of trunk (posterior part)

Axillary tail of breast

## 5. Lateral Group

*Location:*

It lies along the medial side of axillary vein.

*Receive lymph from:*

Upper limb

## 6. Central Group

*Location:*

Located in the axillary fat

*Receives lymph from:*

Anterior, posterior and lateral groups of nodes

## 7. Apical Group

*Location:*

Lies in the apex of the axilla

*Receives lymph from:*

All of the above groups

***Drainage of lymph:*** The lymph from axillary nodes is via efferent vessels ultimately to apical group and then to the neck as follows.

1. By the *subclavian lymph trunk* into the *thoracic duct* (on left side of body)
2. By the subclavian lymph trunk into the *right lymphatic duct* (on right side of body)
3. Direct into the junction of jugulo-subclavian veins in the neck
4. A few efferent lymphatics drain into supraclavicular nodes

> *Significance:* Examination of the axillary lymph nodes is a mandatory part of the evaluation of breast cancer. Involvement of axillary nodes determines the type of surgical and oncologic decisions to be made.

# BREAST

## Extent

- *Horizontally* from the sterna edge to the midaxillary line
- *Vertically* from the 2nd to 6th ribs

- *Axillary tail:* A prolongation of a small part of upper outer quadrant towards the axilla

## Structure

The breast is a modified sweat gland. It begins to develop in the fourth week of intrauterine life from an ectodermal thickening called as *mammary ridge.* Lobulation of the breast occurs after puberty in the females only. Variations in the size of breast are not related to the amount of glandular or secretary tissues. It is determined by the fat content present in individual breast. An extension of breast tissues from the superolateral part towards the axilla is known as axillary tail.

Each mammary gland consists of 15-20 lobes. Each lobe is drained by one *lactiferous duct*. These ducts converge onto the nipple and open individually on its tip. The terminal part of each duct has a dilated sinus in the nipple.

**Nipple** is the conical projection lying slightly below the center of the breast at the level of fourth rib. Smooth muscle fibers are present in the nipple and their contraction leads to the erection of the nipple.

**Areola** is an area of pigmented skin which surrounds the nipple. During pregnancy, large sebaceous glands under the areola may cause small swellings called as *tubercles of Montgomery.*

**Support** to the breast is provided by the *suspensory ligaments of Cooper.* These are the strands of fibrous tissues which connect the dermis of the overlying skin to the ducts of breast and superficial fascia present behind the breast. This fascia is the upward continuation of the membranous layer of the superficial abdominal *fascia Scarpa.* Suspensory ligaments maintain the protuberance of the young breast. However, breast becomes pendulous with the age related atrophy of these ligaments.

**Retromammary space** is a potential space between the pectoral fascia and the breast. It contains loose connective tissues and lies at the base of the breast. It facilitates mobility of breast over the anterior chest wall.

The resting or non-lactating breast usually consists of fibrous and fatty tissue. In pregnant females it enlarges due to an increase and budding of alveoli. Involution of secretary elements occurs when the lactation ceases. After menopause, progressive atrophy of lobes and ducts is the end fate.

The **male breast** resembles the rudimentary female breast having no lobules or alveoli.

***Witch's milk:*** Sometimes infant breast may secrete milk in the first week after birth under the influence of maternal hormones especially estrogen. This fat free fluid is called witch's milk.

## Blood Supply

### *Arterial supply*

1. Lateral thoracic artery (branch of axillary artery) supplies the lateral half.
2. Thoracoacromial artery (branch of axillary artery) supplies the upper outer quadrant.
3. Superior thoracic artery (branch of axillary artery) supplies the upper outer quadrant.
4. Internal thoracic artery (branch of subclavian artery) supplies the medial half.
5. Anterior intercostal arteries (branches of internal thoracic artery) supply the medial half.
6. Posterior intercostals arteries (branches of the thoracic aorta) supply the part overlying the 2$^{nd}$, 3$^{rd}$ and 4$^{th}$ intercostals spaces through the perforating branches.

### *Venous drainage*

The veins converge towards the nipple to form circumareolar plexus. Circumareolar venous plexus drains through two sets of veins:

1. *Superficial set of veins* drains into the internal thoracic vein.
2. *Deep set of veins* drains into
   a. Axillary vein,
   b. Internal thoracic vein and
   c. Posterior intercostal veins.

*Significance:* Posterior intercostal veins drain into the internal vertebral venous plexus. This is one of the important routes of spread of cancer from the breast to the vertebral bodies.

## *Lymph drainage*

### *Major channels*

1. Axillary nodes (mainly anterior) 75%
2. Parasternal nodes
3. Posterior intercostals nodes
4. Superficial lymphatics to opposite breast

### *Minor channels*

1. Supraclavicular nodes
2. Subdiaphragmatic *inferior phrenic* nodes
3. Inferior deep cervical nodes
4. Posterior mediastinal nodes

## *Nerve supply*

The **$4^{th}$-$6^{th}$ intercostals nerves** innervate the breast through their:
1. *Lateral cutaneous* branches and
2. *Anterior cutaneous* branches.

# CLINICAL AND APPLIED INTEGRATION

## Breast Cancer

Breast is an important site of cancer. Its incidence is more than any other type of cancer in females. Spread (metastasis) of breast cancer occurs by the following routes:

1. Direct invasion of the surrounding structures
2. Through blood
3. By lymph channels

### *Incidence of breast cancer*

| | | |
|---|---|---|
| 1. | Upper outer quadrant | 60% |
| 2. | Upper inner quadrant | 12% |
| 3. | Lower outer quadrant | 10% |
| 4. | Lower inner quadrant | 06% |
| 5. | Nipple | 12% |

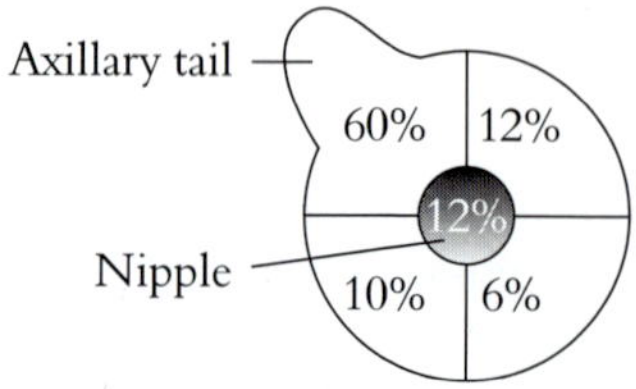

**Mammography** is one of the imaging techniques used to find any mass in the suspected cases of breast cancer. It guides the surgeons for cleavage of a region during removal of breast tissues in cancer cases.

**Lumpectomy** is the local excision of a lump or mass of a breast. It is a breast preserving procedure. Careful and satisfactory lumpectomy by an experience surgeon is a great deal to prevent the patient from a psychological trauma.

**Mastectomy** is the term used for the total excision of the breast. In *simple mastectomy* breast tissues are removed down to the reteromammary space. *Radical mastectomy* implies to the more extensive removal of total breast and axillary tail alongwith the cleavage of the axillary lymph nodes and sometimes the pectoral muscles as well.

## Gynaecomastia

Excessive development of male breast after puberty, even to the functional state, is known as gynaecomastia. It may result due to the imbalance between the estrogen and androgenic hormones. It may occur in cases of sex-chromosomal anomalies e.g. klinefelter syndrome which is an XXY trisomy. More than 40% cases present with gynaecomastia after the onset of puberty in this condition.

# Chapter 13 THE ARM

**ARM** is the region of upper limb which spans between the shoulder bulge and elbow. It is divided into anterior and posterior compartments by the medial and lateral intermuscular septa. These septa arise from the medial and lateral supracondylar lines of the humerus respectively and extend to fuse with the deep fascia of the arm.

### Anterior (Flexor) Compartment Contents

**Muscles:** 1. Biceps brachii 2. Brachialis 3. Coracobrachialis

**Vessels:** 1. Brachial artery 2. Venae comitantes of brachial artery 3. Cephalic vein 4. Basilic vein

**Nerves:** 1. Median nerve 2. Musculocutaneous nerve 3. Ulnar nerve

### Posterior (Extensor) Compartment Contents

**Muscles:** 1. Triceps

**Vessels:** 1. Profunda brachial artery

**Nerves:** 1. Radial nerve 2. Ulnar nerve

## MUSCLES OF THE ARM

### Biceps Brachii

#### *Origin*

1. *Long head* arises from the supraglenoid tubercle.
2. *Short head* arises from the tip of the coracoid's process.

#### *Insertion*

1. *Tendon* insertion is on the radial tuberosity.
2. *Aponeurosis* ( a medial expansion of the tendon) merges with

the deep fascia and then is inserted on the subcutaneous border of the upper end of ulna.

### *Nerve supply*

Musculocutaneous nerve

### *Actions*

1. It is a powerful flexor of elbow joint, but a week flexor of shoulder.
2. Supination of the forearm. It is a powerful supinator when the elbow is flexed.

## Brachialis

### *Origin*

1. Lower half of the front of humerus
2. Medial intermuscular septum

### *Insertion*

1. Coronoid process of ulna
2. Tuberosity of ulna

### *Nerve supply*

1. Musculocutaneous nerve
2. A small part by radial nerve

### *Action*

Flexion of elbow joint

## Coracobrachialis

### *Origin*

Apex of coracoid process

### *Insertion*

Midway on the medial border of humerus

### *Nerve supply*

Musculocutaneous nerve

### *Action*

It is a week flexor and adductor of the shoulder.

## Triceps

### *Origin*

1. Long head—Infraglenoid tubercle
2. Lateral head—Above the radial groove to surgical neck on the back of humerus
3. Medial head—below the radial groove on the back of humerus and both medial and lateral intermuscular septum

### *Insertion*

Upper surface of the olecranon

### *Nerve supply*

Radial nerve

- Branches of radial nerve in the axilla supply the long and medial heads.
- Branches in the radial groove innervate the lateral and medial heads.

### *Action*

Extension of the elbow joint

> The long heads of triceps and biceps lie inferior and superior to the shoulder joint when it is stretched in abduction like *'Guy ropes'* to support and stabilize this joint.

## Radial (Humeral) Groove

It is a spiral groove present on the upper part of anterolateral surface of the humerus. The posterior margin of the groove continues downwards as *lateral supracondylar ridge* which ends at the lateral epicondyle. The less prominent *medial supracondylar ridge* runs down to the medial epicondyle. The lateral and medial supracondylar ridges give attachments to the *medial* and *lateral intermuscular septums* respectively.

### Contents

1. Radial nerve
2. Profunda brachii vessels

> Intramuscular injections given in the triceps by inexperienced hands may damage the contents of the radial groove.

## MUSCULOCUTANEOUS NERVE

### Origin

It emerges from the lateral cord (C5, 6, 7) of brachial plexus.

### Course

- It pierces the coracobrachialis muscle and then descends between biceps and brachialis.
- It then appears at the elbow lateral to the biceps tendon.
- Here it pierces the deep fascia in front of the elbow and continues as lateral cutaneous nerve of the forearm.
- It then courses along the radial border of the forearm from elbow to wrist as the lateral cutaneous nerve of the forearm.

### Branches

1. Muscular branches to Coracobrachialis, biceps, and brachialis.
2. Lateral cutaneous nerve of forearm to the skin over lateral aspect of forearm.

> Musculocutaneous nerve is muscular in the arm and cutaneous in the forearm.

## AXILLARY NERVE

### Origin

It is a branch of the posterior cord of brachial plexus.

### Course

- From the posterior cord it courses posteriorly.
- It then passes through the quadangular space.
- In the quadangular space it divides to terminate into an anterior and a posterior branch.

### Branches

1. Anterior branch to deltoid and shoulder joint
2. Posterior branch to deltoid and teres minor
3. Upper lateral cutaneous nerve of the arm is the continuation of the posterior branch of the axillary nerve which supplies the skin over the upper lateral surface of the arm and lower part of skin over the deltoid.

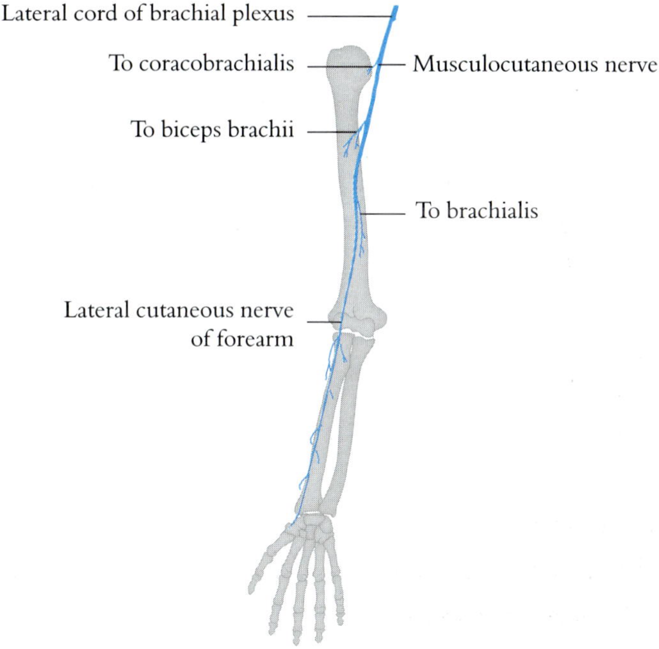


**Fig. 13.1: Origin, course and supply of musculocutaneous nerve**

# CUBITAL FOSSA

It is a triangular fossa which forms the hollow at the front of the elbow.

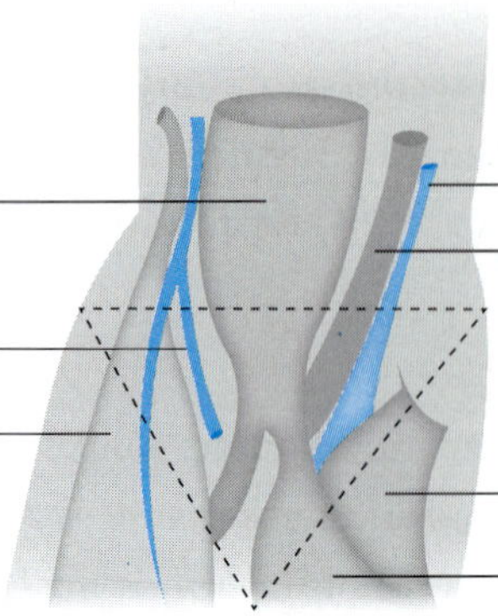


**Fig. 13.2: Boundaries and contents of right cubital fossa**

## *Boundaries*

*Medial Border:* Pronator teres

*Lateral Border:* Brachioradialis

*Base:* An imaginary line drawn between the two epicondyles of the humerus

*Apex:* Directed downwards and formed where pronator teres and brachioradialis meet

*Floor:* Formed by the:

1. Brachialis
2. Supinator

*Roof:* Formed by the:

1. Deep fascia of forearm
2. Bicipital aponeurosis
3. Median cubital vein
4. Medial cutaneous nerve of the forearm

### Contents

(from medial to lateral side)

1. Median nerve
2. Brachial artery
3. Radial and Ulnar arteries
4. Tendon of biceps
5. Radial nerve
6. Posterior interosseous (deep) branch of radial nerve
7. Superficial branch of radial nerve

*Significance:*

1. The brachial artery is palpated here to ascertain the position for placing the stethoscope while taking the blood pressure.
2. Median cubital vein present in the roof is commonly used for:
   a. intravenous injections,
   b. blood sampling and
   c. blood transfusion.

## ELBOW JOINT

### Type

Synovial joint of hinge variety

### Articulating bones

1. Trochlea and capitulum of humerus
2. Trochlear notch of ulna
3. Head of radius

### Stability Factors

#### *1. Ligaments*

a. ***Ulnar (medial) collateral ligament***, a triangular ligament consisting of three bands.

   i. Anterior strongest band passes from medial epicondyle of humerus to sublime tubercle on the coronoid process.

ii. Posterior band joins the sublime tubercle and medial border of olecranon.

iii. Thin middle band connects the two.

b. ***The radial (lateral) collateral ligament*** is also a triangular band. Apex is attached to the lateral epicondyle and base fuses with the annular ligament of the radius.

### *2. Bony Factors*

a. Anterior fossae receiving the head of the humerus and coronoid process of the ulna when the arm is fully flexed.

b. Posterior deep fossa receive the olecranon process of ulna in full extension.

## Nerve Supply

1. Musculocutaneous nerve
2. Median nerve
3. Radial nerve
4. Ulnar nerve

## Movements at Elbow Joint

1. Flexion caused by
   a. Biceps brachii
   b. Coracobrachialis
   c. Brachialis
2. Extension caused by
   a. Triceps

> The range of flexion from the straight extended position is approximately 140° at the elbow joint.

## Carrying Angle

The extended ulna makes an angle of 170° with the humerus. This is called as *carrying angle*. This obliquity of the axis of hinge allows the elbow to fit in the waist when the arm is by the side. It helps to carry the things e.g. a basket. The obliquity of the ulna is more pronounced in females due to the wider pelvis. The carrying angle in females is thus 165°-167°.

## BRACHIAL ARTERY

### *Origin and Course*

- It images at the lower border of teres major.
- It is the continuation of the axillary artery.
- It lies superficial in its course in the arm.
- It courses on the anteromedial aspect of the arm.
- It dips deep in the cubital fossa.
- In the arm it carries venae comitantes.

### *Termination*

- It divides into its terminal branches (radial and ulnar arteries) at the level of neck of the radius.

### *Branches*

1. Profunda brachial artery (largest branch)
2. Radial artery
3. Ulnar artery
4. Superior ulnar collateral artery
5. Inferior ulnar collateral artery
6. Muscular branches to flexor muscles and Nutrient artery to the humerus

> The brachial artery can be palpated at the midpoint of humeral epicondyles. This is the usual site of auscultation for taking blood pressure.

### Profunda Brachii Artery

### *Origin*

- Just below the teres major where it leaves the lower triangular space.
- It runs in the radial groove with radial nerve.
- Pierces the lateral intermuscular septum and divides into two terminal branches.

## *Branches*

1. Radial collateral artery or anterior descending artery
2. Middle collateral artery or posterior descending artery
3. Muscular branches to triceps and deltoid and Nutrient artery to the humerus

## ANASTOMOSIS AROUND ELBOW JOINT

The following arteries participate in the anastomosis around the elbow joint.

### On the Medial Side of Elbow

1. Superior ulnar collateral artery, branch of brachial artery
2. Inferior ulnar collateral artery, branch of brachial artery
3. Anterior ulnar recurrent artery, branch of ulnar artery
4. Posterior ulnar recurrent artery, branch of ulnar artery

### On the Lateral Side of Elbow

1. Anterior radial collateral artery, branch of profunda brachii artery
2. Posterior radial collateral artery, branch of profunda brachii artery
3. Radial recurrent artery, branch of radial artery
4. Interosseous recurrent artery, branch of common interosseous artery

## CLINICAL AND APPLIED INTEGRATION

### Tennis Elbow

This condition is characterized by the inflammation of the lateral epicondyle called as lateral epicondylitis. It occurs due to the repeated stretch and trauma during prolonged use of extensor muscles of the forearm. The site of pain and injury is the common extensor origin at the lateral epicondyle of humerus.

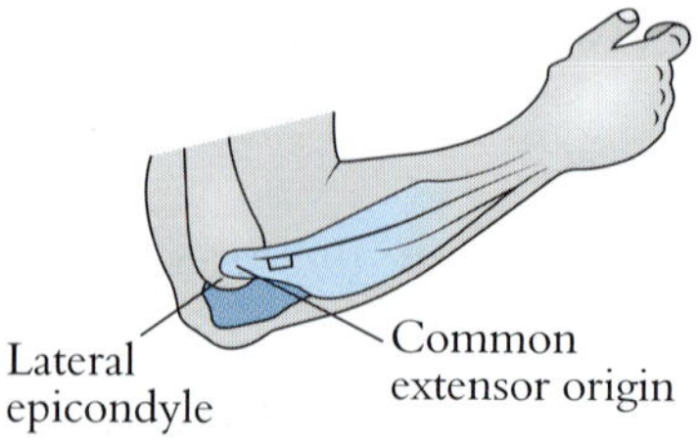


**Fig. 13.3: Tennis elbow**

## Student's Elbow

This condition occurs usually in students when they support their head with the hand and place the flexed elbow on the table during the study hours. Inflammation and pain ensues over the bursa at the triceps insertion due to repeated and prolonged pressure.

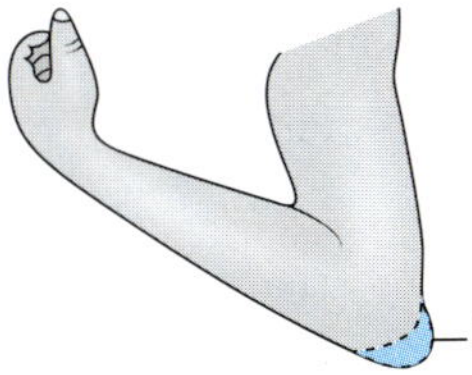


**Fig. 13.4: Student's elbow**

## Golfer's Elbow

This condition is characterized by the inflammation of the medial epicondyle called as medial epicondylitis. It occurs due to the repeated stretch or trauma over the common origin of flexor muscles of the forearm. The site of injury is the common flexor origin at the medial epicondyle of humerus. The individual feels pain and discomfort while flexing the arm.

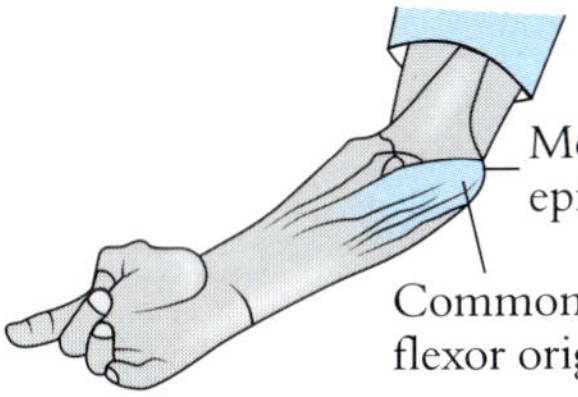


**Fig. 13.5: Golfer's elbow**

Chapter

# 14 THE FOREARM

**FOREARM** is the part of upper limb which spans between the elbow and wrist and connect the arm with the hand. It consists of an anterior (flexor) compartment and a posterior (extensor) compartment.

## Muscles of the Anterior Compartment

The flexor muscles are arranged in two groups:

1. ***Superficial group*** of five muscles
2. ***Deep group*** of three muscles

**Table 14.1: Superficial Flexors of the Forearm**

| Muscle | Origin | Insertion | Nerve Supply | Actions |
|---|---|---|---|---|
| Pronator teres | 1. Medial epicondyle<br>2. Coronoid process of ulna | Middle of lateral surface of shaft of radius | Median nerve (C6, 7) | 1. Pronation of forearm<br>2. Flexion of elbow (weak) |
| Flexor carpi radialis | Medial epicondyle | Base of 2nd and 3rd metacarpals | Median nerve | 1. Flexion of the wrist<br>2. Radial abduction of the wrist |
| Flexor digitorum super-ficialis | 1. Medial epicondyle<br>2. Coronoid process of ulna | | Median nerve | 1. Flexion of proximal inter-phalangeal joint<br>2. Flexion of metacarpo-phalangeal and wrist joint |

| Muscle | Origin | Insertion | Nerve Supply | Actions |
|---|---|---|---|---|
| Palmaris longus | Medial epicondyle | 1. Partially to flexor retina-culum<br>2. Splits to form palmar apone-urosis | Median nerve | Flexion of the wrist (weak) |
| Flexor carpi ulnaris | 1. Medial epicondyle<br>2. Olecranon<br>3. Subcu-taneous border of the ulna | 1. Pisiform bone<br>2. Hamate<br>3. 5th meta-carpal bone | Ulnar nerve (C7, 8) | 1. Flexion of the wrist<br>2. Ulnar adduction of the wrist |

**Table 14.2: Deep Flexors of the Forearm**

| Muscle | Origin | Insertion | Nerve Supply | Actions |
|---|---|---|---|---|
| Flexor digi-torum pro-fundus | 1. Upper 3/4th of ulna (anterior and medial surfaces)<br>2. Interosseous membrane | Insertion is on the distal phalanges of each of the four fingers by a separate tendon. | 1. Ulnar belly: Ulnar nerve<br>2. Radial belly: Median nerve | 1. Flexion of the terminal interph-alageal joints<br>2. It is the muscle of powerful gripping. |

| Muscle | Origin | Insertion | Nerve Supply | Actions |
|---|---|---|---|---|
| Flexor pollicis longus | 1. Anterior surface of shaft of the radius<br>2. Interosseous membrane | Distal phalanx of the thumb | Median nerve (anterior intero-sseous branch) | 1. The only flexor of interphalangeal joint of the thumb<br>2. Flexion of the metacarpophalangeal and capometacarpal joints of the thumb |
| Pronator quadratus | 1. Anteromedial surface of the distal ulna | Lower 1/4th of anterior surface of ulna | Median nerve (anterior intero-sseous branch) | Pronation of forearm (powerful than pronator teres) |

The muscles of the forearm are supplied by three nerves. Each nerve passes between the two heads of a muscle.

1. The median nerve passes between the two heads of pronator teres.
2. The ulnar nerve between the heads of flexor carpi ulnaris.
3. The posterior interosseous (from radial) nerve passes between the two layers of supinator muscle to enter and supply muscles of extensor compartment of forearm.

## Space of Parona

It is a space in front of pronator quadrates and deep to the long flexor tendons of the fingers. The space is limited proximally by the oblique origin of flexor digitorum superficialis. Proximal parts of flexor synovial sheaths protrude in it. Therefore, it may get involved in the proximal extension of synovial sheath infections.

## Muscles of the Posterior Compartment

Dozens of extensors occupy the posterior(extensor) compartment of the forearm. These muscles are arranged in the following groups:

### *1. Upper group*

a. Anconeus (superficial)

b. Supinator (Deep)

### *2. Lateral group*

a. Brachioradialis

b. Ext. Carpi radialis longus

c. Ext. Carpi radialis brevis

### *3. Posterior group*

a. Ext. Digitorum

b. Ext. Carpi ulnaris

c. Ext. Digiti minimi

### *4. Lower group*

a. Abductor policis longus

b. Ext. Policis longus

c. Ext. Policis brevis

### *5. Index group*

a. Ext. Indicis

**Table 14.3: Muscles of Posterior Compartment of Forearm**

| Muscle | Origin | Insertion | Nerve Supply | Actions |
|---|---|---|---|---|
| 1. Anconeus | Lateral epicondyle | 1. Olecranon process<br>2. Ulnar shaft | Radial nerve | Extension and abduction of ulna in the pronation |

| Muscle | Origin | Insertion | Nerve Supply | Actions |
|---|---|---|---|---|
| 2. Supinator | 1. Lateral epicondyle<br>2. Lateral ligament<br>3. Annular ligament | Between anterior and posterior oblique lines of radius on its lateral surface | Posterior inteross-eous nerve | Supination when the elbow is extended |
| 3. Brachio-radialis | Lat. Supraco-ndylar ridge of humerus | Base of radial styloid | Radial nerve | Flexion of elbow joint |
| 4. Ext. carpi radialis longus | Lat. Supraco-ndylar ridge of humerus | 2nd metacarpal base | Radial nerve | 1. Extension and abduction of wrist<br>2. Used in making fist |
| 5. Ext. carpi radialis brevis | Common ext. origin | 3rd metacarpal base | Posterior inteross-eous nerve | 1. Wrist extensor<br>2. Used in making fist |
| 6. Ext. digitorum | Common extensor origin | Four tendons form extensor expansion, inserted into respective medial four phalanges. | Posterior inteross-eous nerve | Extend the proximal medial four phalanges |
| 7. Ext. digiti minimi | Common extensor origin | Joins and forms extensor expansion to be inserted on the dorsum of little finger | Posterior inteross-eous nerve | Extend the proximal phalanx of little finger |

| Muscle | Origin | Insertion | Nerve Supply | Actions |
|---|---|---|---|---|
| 8. Ext. carpi ulnaris | Common extensor origin | Base of 5th metacarpal | Posterior inteross-eous nerve | Extensor and adductor of the wrist |
| 9. Abductor pollicis longus | From the back of ulna, radius and interosseous membrane | Two slips of tendon attached to the base of 1st metacarpal and trapezium | Posterior inteross-eous nerve | 1. Extends the thumb at carpo-metacar-pal joint. Laterally displaces thumb<br>2. Assists in abduction and flexion of the wrist |
| 10. Ext. pollicis brevis | Radius and adjacent interosseous membrane | Base of proximal phalanx of thumb | Posterior inteross-eous nerve | Extends car-pometacarpal and metacar-pophalangeal joints |
| 11. Ext. pollicis longus | From ulna distal to abd. Pollicis longus | Base of the distal phalanx of thumb | Posterior inteross-eous nerve | 1. Extends the terminal phalanx of thumb<br>2. Assists extension and abduction of wrist |
| 12. Ext. indicis | From ulna distal to ext. pollicis longus | Joins the dorsal expansion of index finger | Posterior inteross-eous nerve | Extends the little finger |

Pointing by the index finger is done by the extensor indicis muscle.

## Extensor Retinaculum

It is a 2.5 cm broad fascial band lying obliquely across the extensor surface of the wrist.

1. It is proximally attached to the anterolateral border of the radius just above the styloid process.
2. Distally, it is attached to the pisiform and triquetral bones.
3. Fibrous septa from its deep surface extend to radius and ulna and divide the extensor tunnel into six compartments, which are:
    a. Most lateral compartment. Transmits tendons of:
        i. abductor pollicis longus
        ii. extensor pollicis brevis
    b. Lateral surface to dorsal tubercle. Transmits tendon of:
        i. extensor carpi radialis longus
        ii. extensor carpi radialis brevis
    c. Groove on ulnar side of radial tubercle lodges tendon of:
        i. extensor pollicis longus
    d. Between the groove and ulnar border of radius pass
        i. four tendons of extensor digitorum
        ii. extensor indicis
    e. Compartment over the radioulnar joint conveys the tendon of:
        i. extensor digiti minimi
    f. Groove near the styloid process of ulna transmits:
        i. extensor carpi ulnaris

All the tendons are invested in a separate synovial sheath except the four tendons of extensor digitorum and a tendon of extensor indicis which share a common sheath.

### *Other structures passing behind the extensor retinaculum*

1. Posterior cutaneous branch of ulnar nerve
2. Superficial branch of radial nerve
3. The cephalic vein
4. The basilic vein

## Anatomical Snuffbox

It is a concavity on the radial side of the wrist between the tendons of the thumb.

### *Boundaries*

*Medial:* Extensor pollicis longus tendon

*Lateral:* Extensor pollicis brevis and abductor pollicis longus tendons

*Roof:* Skin, Fascia, Cephalic vein and Cutaneous branches of radial nerve

*Floor (from proximal to distal):*

1. Styloid process of radius
2. Scaphoid
3. Trapezium
4. Base of 1st metacarpal

### *Contents*

Radial artery

*Significance:*

1. One of the sites for the palpation of radial pulse
2. Site for the palpation of scaphoid bone
3. Commonest site for the formation of fistula for hemodialysis in renal failure patients

## RADIAL ARTERY

- Radial artery originates in the cubital fossa as the direct continuation of brachial artery.
- It passes distally medial to the biceps tendon to the lower end of radius.
- It lies between the brachioradialis tendon laterally and flexor carpi radialis tendon medially.
- Bed is formed by supinator, pronator teres, flexor digitorum superficialis, flexor pollicis longus, the pronator quadrates, and the lower end of radius.
- In the middle third of forearm, radial nerve lies lateral to it.
- It disappears beneath the tendons of abductor pollicis longus and extensor pollicis brevis.

- It crosses the anatomical snuff box and continues in the hand as the deep palmar arch.

### *Branches*

1. Radial recurrent artery
2. Palmar carpal branch
3. Dorsal carpal branch
4. Branch to superficial palmar arch
5. First dorsal metacarpal artery
6. Radialis indicis artery
7. Princeps pollicis artery
8. Deep palmar artery, a terminal branch, which continues in the deep palmar arch
9. Muscular branches

> It is subcutaneous distally over the radius, so is commonly used to feel and count the radial pulse.

## ULNAR ARTERY

- It originates in the cubital fossa as the largest terminal branch of brachial artery.
- It courses deep to pronator teres, flexor digitorum superficialis and median nerve.
- It then runs on flexor digitorum profundus with ulnar nerve to its medial side.
- Passes down into the palm in front of flexor retinaculum and continues as superficial palmar arch.

### *Branches*

1. Common interosseous artery
2. Anterior ulnar recurrent artery
3. Posterior ulnar recurrent artery
4. Palmar and dorsal carpal arteries
5. Superficial palmar branch
6. Deep palmar branch joins deep palmar arch
7. Muscular branches

> Ulnar pulsation can be felt on the radial side of the tendon of flexor carpi ulnaris above the pisiform bone.

## RADIAL NERVE (C5,6,7,8,T1)

### *Origin*

It is the direct continuation of the posterior cord of brachial plexus. It is the largest branch of brachial plexus. It is the nerve of the extensor compartment of the arm and forearm.

### *Course*

1. It descends between the long and medial heads of the triceps.
2. It spirals back around the shaft of humerus through the radial groove and pierces the lateral intermusclar septum.
3. In the lower arm, it descends in the slit between the brachialis and brachioradialis.
4. It courses down in the flexor compartment of the forearm and after winding a round the lower end of the radius, passes through the anatomical snuff box to reach the back of the hand.

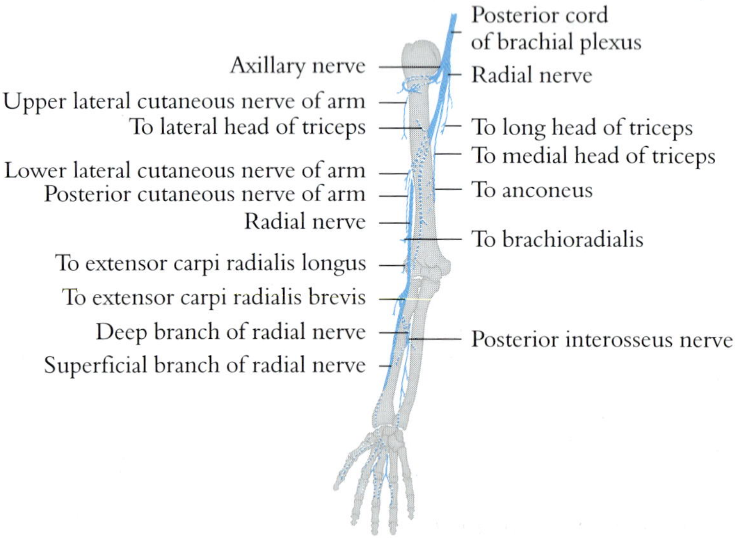


**Fig .14.1: Origin, course and supply of radial nerve**

## Branches

### In the axilla

Posterior cutaneous nerve of the arm

### In the upper arm

1. Posterior cutaneous nerve of forearm
2. Lower lateral cutaneous nerve of arm
3. Muscular branches to triceps, brachioradialis, extensor carpi and a small part of brachialis
4. Articular branch to elbow joint

### In the forearm

1. Deep branch to supinator, extensor compartment muscles and abductor pollicis longus
2. Superficial branch gives no supply in forearm

### In the hand

Superficial branch supplies the skin over the lateral side of the dorsum of hand and lateral 3 ½ fingers.

# ULNAR NERVE (C8 AND T1)

## Origin

It is the direct continuation of the medial cord of brachial plexus.

## Course

1. It courses down between the axillary artery and vein behind the medial cutaneous nerve of the forearm.
2. It pierces the meial intermuscular septum and descends in the groove on the back of medial epicondyle.
3. It enters the flexor compartment of the forearm after passing between the two heads of flexor carpi ulnaris.
4. It courses on the flexor digitorum profundus along with the ulnar artery on its lateral side, and the two cross the flexor retinaculum lateral to the pisiform bone. Here it divides into superficial and deep branches.
5. It ends by supplying the adductor pollicis.

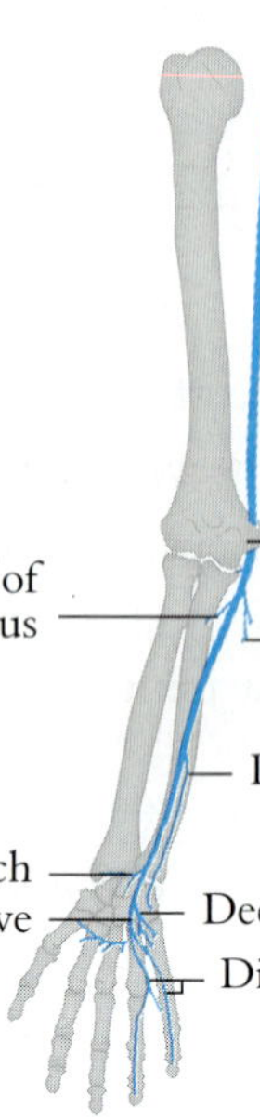


**Fig .14.2: Origin, course and supply of ulnar nerve**

## *Branches*

### *In the axilla*

No branch

### *In the upper arm*

Elbow joint

### *In the forearm*

1. Muscular branches to flexor carpi ulnaris and medial head of Flexor digitorum profundus
2. Posterior cutaneous branch with cutaneous supply in the hand
3. Wrist joint

### *In the hand*

1. Musles of hypothenar eminence
2. Adductor pollicis

3. 3rd and 4th lumbricals (medial two)
4. Interossei
5. Skin of dorsum of medial 1 ½ fingers
6. Palmar digital branches to medial 1 ½ fingers
7. Articular branches to the joints of hand

## MEDIAN NERVE ( C5,6,7,8,T1)

### *Origin*

Roots from lateral and medial cords of brachial plexus

### *Course*

1. It leaves the axilla and in the middle of the arm it crosses in front of the brachial artery.
2. At the elbow it lies medial to the brachial artery beneath the bicipital aponeurosis.
3. In the forearm, it passes between the two heads of pronator teres and courses below the fibrous arch of the flexor digitorum superficialis.
4. It then courses through the carpal tunnel into the hand.

### *Branches*

#### *In the axilla*

No branch in the axilla

#### *In the upper arm*

No branch

#### *In the forearm*

1. Muscular branches to palmaris longus, pronator quadratus, flexor carpi radialis, flexor digitorum superficialis, flexor digitorum profundus (lateral head), flexor pollicis longus
2. Anterior introsseous nerve
3. Articular branches to elbow and wrist joint

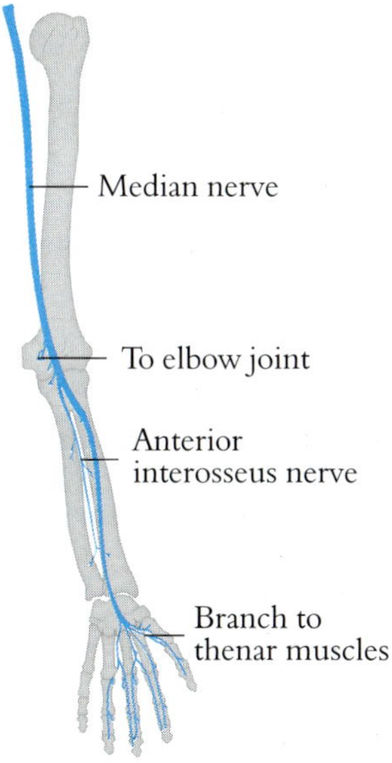


**Fig 14.3: Origin, course and supply of median nerve**

### *In the hand*

1. Branches to three thenar muscles
2. 1st and 2nd lumbricals (medial two)
3. Palmar cutaneous branch
4. Palmar digital branches to lateral 3 ½ fingers

# RADIOULNAR JOINTS

## Proximal Radioulnar Joint

### *Type*

Uniaxial synovial joint of pivot variety

### *Articulating bones*

1. Head of radius
2. Radial notch of ulna

### *Ligaments*

1. Annular ligament, formed by the fibro-osseous ring lined internally by hyaline cartilage
2. Lateral ligament which merges with the annular ligament
3. Quadrate ligament

### *Capsule*

Lined by synovial membrane and attached to the annular ligament

### *Nerve supply*

Same as that of elbow joint i.e. branches from musculocutaneous, median, radial and ulnar nerves

## Distal Radioulnar Joint

### *Type*

Uniaxial, synovial joint of pivot variety

### *Articulating bones*

1. Head of ulna
2. Ulnar notch of the radius

### *Articulating disc*

This is a triangular fibrocartilaginous disc. The base is attached to the ulnar notch of radius and the apex to a fossa at the styloid process of ulna.

### *Nerve supply*

1. Anterior interosseous nerve
2. Posterior interosseous nerve

## Movements at Radioulnar Joints

The movements occurring at this joint and their characteristic features are:

1. Supination
2. Pronation
    - In full supination, the radius lies laterally and parallel to ulna.
    - In full pronation, the shaft of the radius crosses the ulna anteriorly and its lower end then lies medially.
    - Supination is the more powerful act.

Chapter

# 15 THE WRIST AND HAND

**WRIST and HAND** are the most distal and terminal regions of the upper limb and comprise the wrist joint, dorsum and palm of the hand.

## WRIST JOINT

- Biaxial type of synovial joint is also called as radiocarpal joint.
- Articulating bones are the concave distal surface of radius, scaphoid, lunate and triquetral bones.
- The articulating disc of fibrocartilage separates the wrist joint from the radioulnar joint.
- A capsule surrounds the joint and is thickened to form the collateral, palmar and dorsal ligaments.
- The wrist normally remains in a state of slight adduction and extension.
- Nerve Supply:
  1. Anterior interosseous branch of median nerve
  2. Posterior interosseous branch of radial nerve

### Movements

*Flexion:* Caused by

1. Flexor carpi radialis
2. Flexor carpi ulnaris
3. Assisted by palmaris longus and flexors of fingers and thumb. Range of flexion is 80°.

*Extension:*

1. Extensor carpi radialis longus
2. Extensor carpi radialis brevis
3. Extensor carpi ulnaris
4. Assisted by extensors of fingers and thumb. Range is 60°.

*Adduction:*

1. Flexor carpi radialis
2. Extensor carpi radialis longus
3. Extensor carpi radialis brevis
4. Assisted by abductor pollicis longus. Range of movements is limited to 15° due to the styloid process.

*Abduction:*

1. Flexor carpi ulnaris
2. Extensor carpi ulnaris. Range is 45°.

*Circumduction:* The above four movements occurring in a proper sequence produces circumduction.

## FLEXOR RETINACULUM

It is a fibrous band lying in front of the carpus, distal to the distal skin crease of the wrist.

- It is 2-3 cm in width and length.
- *Medially* it is attached to the hook of hamate and pisiform.
- *Laterally* to the tubercle of scaphoid and the trapezium
- *Above,* it is continuous with the fascia of forearm and *below* with the palmar aponeurosis.

### Structures Passing Beneath the Flexor Retinaculum: (Medial to Lateral)

1. Tendon of flexor carpi radialis
2. Tendon of flexor pollicis longus
3. Median nerve
4. Four tendons of flexor digitorum superficialis, in two rows anteriorly
5. Four tendons of flexor digitorum profundus, in one row dorsal to superficialis tendons

The tendon of flexor carpi radialis and flexor pollicis longus are enclosed in their own synovial sheath separately. The digitorum tendons of both superficial and deep group collectively share a common sheath which they invaginate from radial side. The blood supply of these tendons gains access from the open radial side.

## Structures Passing Above or Superficial to the Flexor Retinaculum: (Medial To Lateral)

1. Ulnar artery
2. Ulnar nerve
3. Palmar cutaneous branch of ulnar nerve
4. Palmaris longus tendon
5. Palmar cutaneous branch of median nerve
6. Superficial palmar branch of radial artery

## Carpal Tunnel

It is a fibro-osseous canal, which lies between the flexor retinaculum and carpal bones. This tunnel is the result of deep anterior concavity of the carpus.

*Contents:*

All the structures passing deep to the flexor retinaculum

### *Canal of guyon*

Is the slender band of fascia which encloses the ulnar artery and ulnar nerve. It lies lateral to the pisiform bone in front of flexor retinaculum. Occasionally ulnar nerve is compressed here.

## PALMAR APONEUROSIS

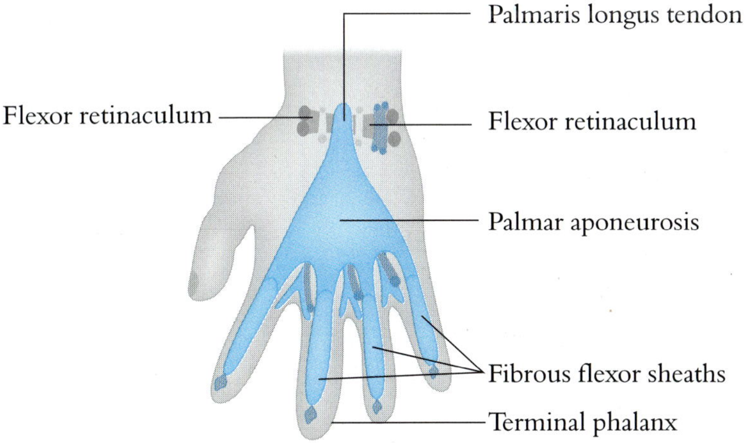


**Fig. 15.1: Palmar aponeurosis**

It is the thickening of the deep fascia of the central region of the palm of hand.

- It is triangular in shape with the apex directed upwards.
- It is continuous proximally with the flexor retinaculum and on either side by the fascia of the thenar and hypothenar eminences.
- Distally it widens and divides into four slips, one for each finger.
- The main part of each digital slip divides into two diverging bands which are inserted into the transverse metacarpal ligament and the fibrous flexor sheath.
- Its fibers are continuous with the fibers of the Palmaris longus tendon.
- It fixes the skin of the palm and thus improves the grip.
- It protects the underlying structures lying deep to it i.e., superficial palmar arch, long flexor tendons, superficial branch of ulnar nerve, and terminal part of median nerve.

## THENAR EMINENCE

It is the horizontal protrusion at the proximal part of the palm which extends from the base of the thumb to the middle of the palm. It is produced by the three short muscles of the thumb i.e., abductor pollicis brevis, flexor pollicis brevis, and opponens pollicis. All these muscles take origin from the flexor retinaculum.

### Muscles of the Thenar Eminence

1. Abductor pollicis brevis
2. Flexor pollicis brevis
3. Opponens pollicis

### Long Tendons of the Thumb

1. Flexor pollicis longus
2. Extensor pollicis longus
3. Extensor pollicis brevis

**Table 15-1: Muscles of the Thenar Eminence**

| Muscle | Origin | Insertion | Nerve supply | Action |
|---|---|---|---|---|
| Abd. Pollicis brevis | 1. Flex or Retinaculum<br>2. Scaphoid | 1. Proximal phalanx base<br>2. Ext. pollicis longus | Median nerve | 1. Thumb abduction<br>2. Assists extension |
| Flex. Pollicis brevis | 1. Superficial head: Flexor Retinaculum and trapezium.<br>2. Deep head: Trapezoid and capitate | Base of proximal phalanx of thumb | Median nerve | Flexion of thumb |
| Oppo-nens pollicis | 1. Flex or Retinaculum and trapezium | Radial border of the 1st metacarpal bone (of the thumb) | Median nerve | Opposition by making the thumbnail parallel to the nail of opposing finger |
| Adductor pollicis | 1. Transverse head: palmar border of 3rd metacarpal<br>2. Oblique head: bases of 2nd and 3rd metacarpals and the capitate | Base of the proximal phalanx of thumb.<br>Ulnar sesamoid of the thumb. | Deep branch of ulnar nerve | Proximation of the thumb to the index finger |

## Movements of the Thumbs

### *Flexion*

1. Flexor pollicis longus
2. Flexor pollicis brevis

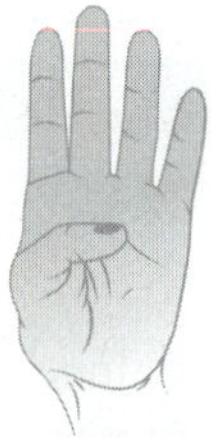


### *Extension*

1. Extensor pollicis longus
2. Extensor pollicis brevis

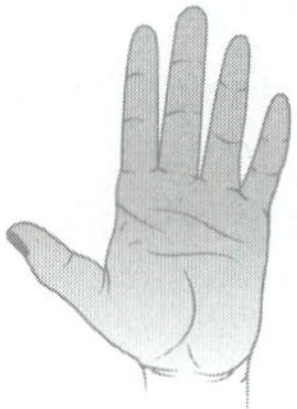


### *Palmar abduction*

1. Abductor pollicis brevis

### *Radial abduction*

1. Abductor pollicis longus

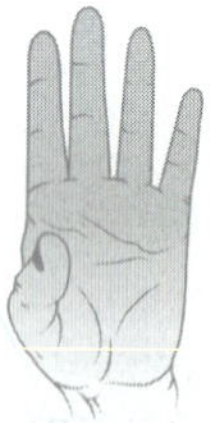


### *Adduction*

1. Adductor pollicis
2. Flexor pollicis brevis

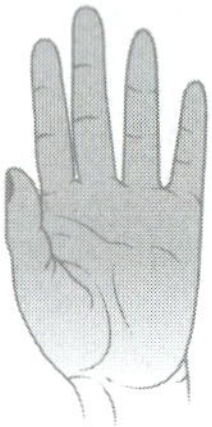


### *Opposition*

1. Opponens pollicis

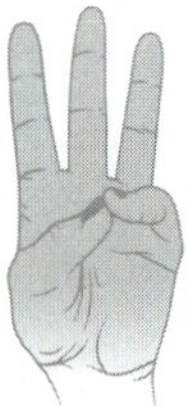


### *Circumduction*

Combined action of all the muscles

## HYPOTHENAR EMINENCE

It is a vertical protrusion present at the ulnar side of palm extending from the base of the little finger to the proximal limit of the palm. It is formed by three short muscles of the little finger.

**Table 15-2: Muscles of the Hyothenar Eminence**

| Muscle | Origin | Insertion | Nerve supply | Action |
|---|---|---|---|---|
| Abductor digiti minimi | Pisiform bone<br>Flexor Carpi ulnaris tendon | Ulnar side of base of proximal phalanx<br>Extensor expansion | Deep branch ulnar nerve | All three muscles assist to grip large objects;<br>Help to cup the palm |
| Flexor digiti minimi brevis | Hook of hamate<br>Flexor retinaculum | Ulnar side of base of proximal phalanx | | |
| Opponens digiti minimi | Hook of Hamate<br>Flexor retinaculum | Ulnar border of 5th metacarpal bone | | |

## LUMBRICALS

All the four lumbricals originate from each tendon of flexor digitorum profundus.

They all pass on the radial side of the parent tendon.

Each is inserted into the extensor expansion on the dorsum of hand.

Two lumbricals on the ulnar side are innervated by ulnar nerve and the two on the radial side are innervated by median nerve.

Lumbricals supplied by ulnar nerve are bicipital while those supplied by the median nerve are unicipital.

Lumbricals have no bony attachment hence they are very mobile.

They act as proprioception bridge between flexor and extensor tendons and, therefore, adjust the position of the joints of fingers when the hand is in use.

They also extend the interphalangeal joints when working with extensors.

## INTEROSSEOUS MUSCLES

### Table 15-3: Comparison of Palmar and Dorsal Interossei

| Palmar interossei | Dorsal inteossei |
|---|---|
| Arise from one metacarpal bone | Arise from two adjacent metacarpal bones |
| Small in size | Larger in size |
| Can be seen from palmar aspect only | Can be seen from both palmar and dorsal aspects |
| No palmar interosseous of middle finger<br>(therefore, no adduction on itself) | Dorsal interossei present on either side of middle finger |
| Inserted into the extensor expansion | Also inserted into the extensor expansion |
| Less powerful than dorsal interossei | More powerful than palmar interossei |
| Supplied by deep branch of ulnar nerve | Also supplied by deep branch of ulnar nerve |
| Adduct the little, ring and index fingers towards the midline (action-PAD) | Abduct all four fingers away from the midline (action-DAB) |

## SUPERFICIAL PALMAR ARCH

- It is an arterial arcade which lies in the palmar compartment just deep to the palmar aponeurosis.
- It is the direct continuation of the ulnar artery.
- It commences from the distal border of flexor retinaculum.
- It is usually an incomplete arch.
- It may be complete when it becomes continuous with the superficial branch of radial artery.

- It lies across the central part of palm at the level of distal border of the outstretched thumb.

### *Branches*

(Emerging from the convexity of the arch)

1. One palmar digital artery to the ulnar side
2. Three common digital arteries
3. Proper palmar digital branches of above arteries which supply the adjacent parts of the fingers except the thumb and the radial side of the index finger (both are supplied by the radial artery)
4. Palmar digital arteries anastomose with the dorsal digital arteries and supply the nail beds and distal part of the dorsum of hand.

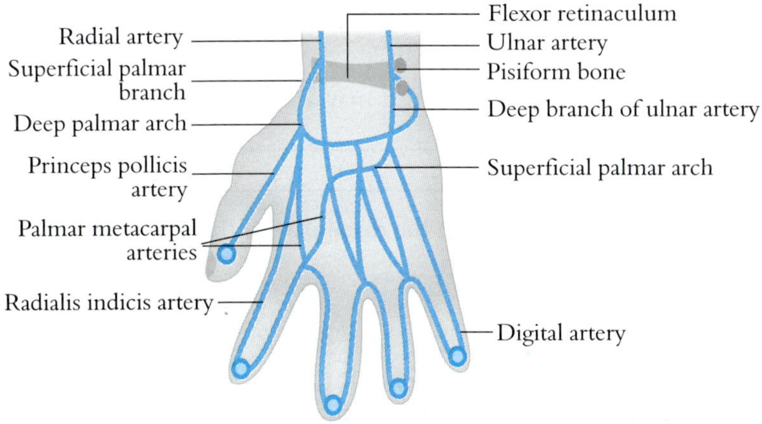


**Fig. 15.2: The superficial and deep palmar arches**

## DEEP PALMAR ARCH

- It is an arterial arcade running across the palm.
- It is formed by the anastomosis of terminal branch of radial artery with the deep branch of ulnar artery.
- It lies one cm proximal to the superficial arch.
- It is usually a complete arch.

### *Branches*

1. Three palmar metacarpal arteries

2. They anastomose with the common palmar digital branches of the superficial arch.
3. Perforating branches anastomose with the dorsal metacarpal arteries.
4. Branches of anterior carpal arch also anastomose with the deep arch.

## PALMAR SPACES

These are the spaces lying beneath the palmar aponeurosis. These spaces are separated from each other by two septums extending down from the ulnar and radial borders of the palmar aponeurosis. These potential spaces are called :

1. Hypothenar space lying on the ulnar side of the palm
2. Mid-palmar space present in the middle part
3. Thenar space on the radial side

In case of infection of the hand, pus may accumulate in these spaces.

## WEB SPACES

These are three spaces lying in the distal part of the palm between the bases of four fingers.

### *Contents*

1. Superficial transverse ligament of the palm
2. Deep transverse ligament of the palm
3. Digital vessels
4. Digital nerves
5. Tendons of the interossei
6. Tendons of the lumbricals
7. Loose fibrofatty tissue

## PULP SPACES

These are the spaces present on the palmar side of the tips of fingers and thumb. They are limited proximally by the firm adherence of the skin of distal flexion cease to the underlying tissues. Due to these adhesion, infection cannot spread upwards along the fingers. Infection of the pulp spaces may occlude the digital vessels coursing through it and may result in the necrosis of the end of distal phalanx.

## GRIP OF HAND OR GRASP

Holding an object in the hand by an individual is called grip. There are many types of grips, each serves a different function and purpose.

### Types of Grips

1. **Power grip:** It is caused by the long flexors of the fingers and the opponens pollicis. The grip is more firm and tight when wrist extensors contract simultaneously.
2. **Hook grip:** In this grip, only long flexors are in action e.g. carrying a basket or a briefcase. Wrist extensors and thumb opposition is usually not required in this grip.
3. **Precision or perfect grip:** It is the finest type of grip. It deals with the holding of very small objects e.g. holding a needle or a pen etc. It requires a very stable wrist and firm opposition of thumb to the index finger. Small muscles of the hand especially the lumbricals are of prime importance to adjust the position of fingers because they are the proprioceptive bridges between the flexors and extensors of the fingers.
4. **Pinch:** It is the crude but firm form of precise grip. However, pinch can be observed as a forced entanglement of an object between the thumb and index finger. This type of grip when applied on any body part may elicit pain.

### Factors Determining the Force of Grip

1. Small, multiple adjustable bones
2. Thenar and hypothenar eminences and their position
3. Hollowness or cupping in the mid palm
4. Double layer of forearm flexors with dual innervations by median and ulnar nerves
5. Additional muscles for thumb, index, and little fingers
6. Palmar creases and flexor creases

Grip is weak when the wrist is flexed. This maneuver is usually used to open the tightly closed fingers of an individual or to recover an object from his firm and powerful grip.

## CLINICAL AND APPLIED INTEGRATION

### Bennett's Fracture

It is an oblique fracture of the base of 1st metacarpal (of thumb). It is caused when the thumb is forcefully abducted. The fracture also extends and runs into the carpometacarpal joint.

### Dupuytren's Contracture

It is the contraction of the palmar aponeurosis and its digital strips due to inflammation leading to the fixed flexion of fingers on the ulnar part of the palmar aponeurosis. The ring and little fingers are mostly involved. The contracture usually affects the men over the age of 50 years. Surgical excision of the contracture is done to relieve the contracture.

### Carpal Tunnel Syndrome

It occurs due to the compression of the tendons or the median nerve by their synovial sheaths. It may be the result of edema, inflammation, or infection of its contents. Mostly the median nerve is affected. The characteristic features include sensory loss over the skin of lateral three and half digits. Opposition of the thumb is also lost. The individual is unable to button his shirt. The compression may be released by partial or complete division of the flexor retinaculum surgically.

### Mallet Finger or Baseball Finger

The insertion of the extensor tendon into the base of the distal phalanx is ruptured as a result of sudden hyperextension in an attempt to catch the balls. It is usually seen in the baseball players. In this condition partial permanent flexion of the terminal phalanx of a finger is caused by an object striking the end or back of the finger due to the rupture of the extensor tendon on its attachment.

### Felon

It refers to the infection of any one pulp spaces of the finger. It is also called as whitlow. The pulp space of the fingers is a closed space. Any injury, usually a pin prick may lead to the purulent infection of the pulp of the distal phalanx of the affected finger. However, the proximal spread of the infection is limited by the firm attachment of the distal crease of the phalanx.

Chapter

# 16 MISCELLANEOUS

## RADIOGRAPHS OF THE UPPER LIMB

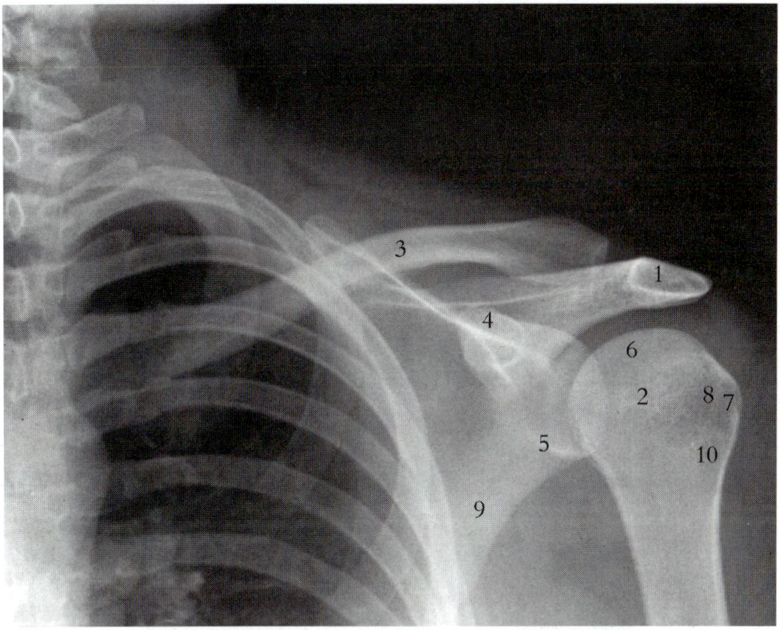


**Fig. 16.1: X-ray ( AP view ) of the shoulder, showing the bony features of the shoulder girdle**

1. Acromion 2. Anatomical neck of humerus 3. Clavicle 4. Coracoid process 5. Glenoid cavity 6. Greater tuberosity 7. Head of humerus 8. Lesser tubercle 9. Lateral border of the scapula 10. Surgical neck of humerus

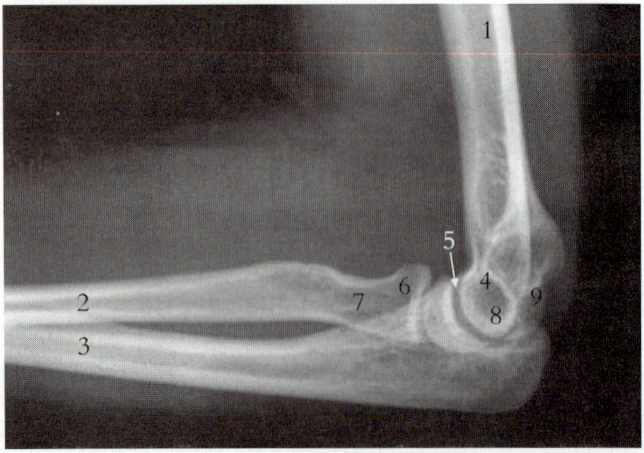


**Fig. 16.2: X-ray (lateral view) showing articulating bones of elbow joint**

1. Humerus 2. Radius 3. Ulna 4. Capitulum of humerus 5. Coronoid process of ulna 6. Head of radius 7. Neck of radius 8. Trochlear notch of ulna 9. Tuberosity of radius

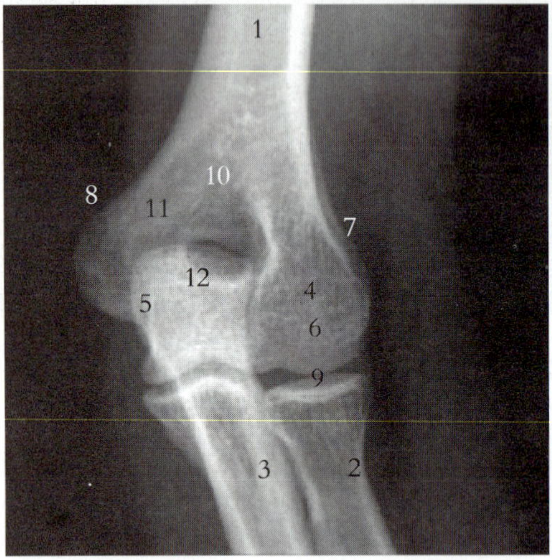


**Fig. 16.3: X-ray (posterior view) showing the bony landmarks of elbow joint**

1. Humerus 2. Radius 3. Ulna 4. Capitulum of humerus 5. Coronoid process of ulna 6. Head of radius 7. Lateral epicondyle of humerus

8. Medial epicondyle of humerus 9. Neck of radius 10. Olecranon fossa of humerus 11. Olecranon of ulna 12. Trochlea of humerus

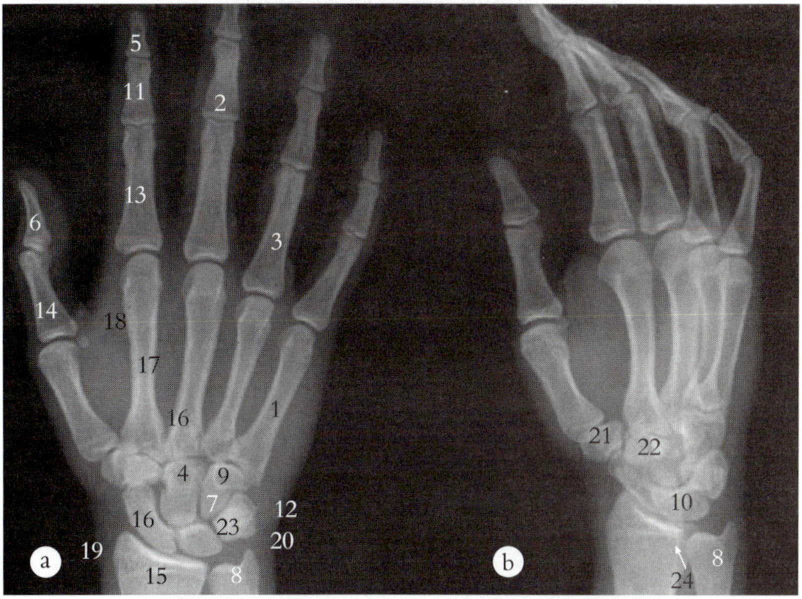


**Fig. 16.4: X-ray showing the bones of the hand and wrist (a) dorsal view (b) oblique view**

1. Fifth metacarpal 2. Base of middle phalanx of middle finger 3. Base of proximal phalanx of ring finger 4. Capitate 5. Distal phalanx of index finger 6. Distal phalanx of thumb 7. Hamate 8. Head of ulna 9. Hook of hamate 10. Lunate 11. Middle phalanx of index finger 12. Pisiform 13. Proximal phalanx of index finger 14. Proximal phalanx of thumb 15. Radius 16. Scaphoid 17. Second metacarpal 18. Sesamoid bone 19. Styloid process of radius 20. Styloid process of ulna 21. Trapezium 22. Trapezoid 23. Triquetral 24. Ulnar notch of radius

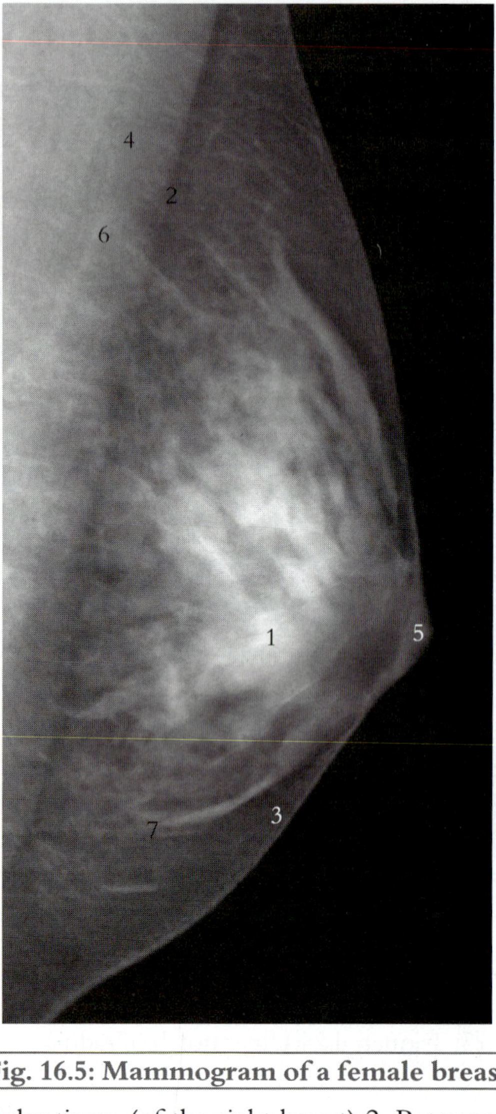


**Fig. 16.5: Mammogram of a female breast**

1. Fibroglandular tissue (of the right breast) 2. Retromammary space 3. Skin 4. Pectoralis major muscle 5. Nipple and areola 6. Vessel 7. Cooper's ligament

## COMMON SITES OF FRACTURES AND DISLOCATIONS OF UPPER LIMB WITH THE RELATED NERVE INJURY

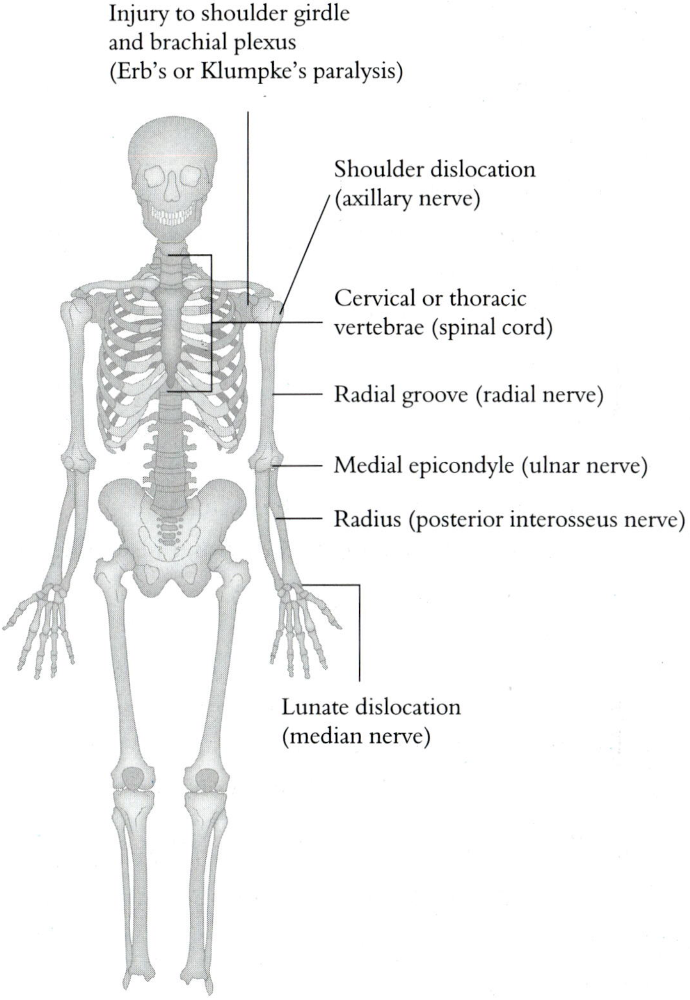


**Fig. 16.6: Schematic diagram showing the common side of fracture and nerve injury of upper limb**

## SURFACE ANATOMY

### Axillary Artery

It lies on a straight line joining the:

1. Mid-clavicular point,
2. Inferior limit of lateral wall of axilla where it terminates.

### Brachial Artery

It lies between the points located:

1. At the termination of axillary artery i.e., at the inferior limit of lateral wall of the axilla,
2. In the cubital fossa, in front of elbow, medial to biceps tendon.

### Radial Artery

It courses between the

1. Just medial to the biceps tendon in the cubital fossa,
2. Medial to the styloid process of the radius,
3. Joins the two points by a line slightly convex laterally.

### Ulnar Artery

It courses between the

1. Medial to biceps tendon in the cubital fossa:
2. Radial side of pisiform bone in the wrist,
3. Joins the two points by a line slightly convex medially.

### Superficial Palmar Arch

It is marked as a distally convex line by joining the points on the

1. Pisiform bone,
2. Hook of hamate,
3. Distal border of thenar eminence vertically in alignment with the cleft between the middle and index finger.

### Deep Palmar Arch

It is slightly convex and lies just distal to the bases of the metacarpal bones, ½ inch (1.3cm) proximal to superficial palmar arch.

## Axillary Nerve

Axillary nerve (or its anterior branch) lies on a horizontal line on the deltoid which lies:

1. 2 cm above the midpoint between the tip of acromion and deltoid tuberosity or
2. Four fingers breadth distal to the tip of acromion.

## Musculocutaneous

It lies on a line joining the:

1. Point located 3 cm above the termination of axillary artery and,
2. 2 cm above the bend of the elbow.

## Median Nerve

It lies on the line joining the points

1. Lateral to the commencement of brachial artery in the upper half of the arm,
2. Medial to the brachial artery in the bend of elbow (cubital fossa);
3. In front of the wrist over the tendon of Palmaris longus.

## Radial Nerve

It lies on a line joining the points on the:

1. Inferior limit of lateral axillary wall,
2. Junction of upper 1/3rd and lower 2/3rds of a line extending between deltoid tuberosity and lateral epicondyle,
3. Front of cubital fossa, 1 cm lateral to biceps tendon,
4. Junction of upper 2/3rd and lower 1/3rd of lateral border of forearm,
5. The anatomical snuff box.

## Ulnar Nerve

It lies on a line joining the points on the:

1. Lower limit of lateral axillary wall,
2. Middle of the medial border of arm,
3. Behind the medial epicondyle,
4. Lateral to the pisiform bone.

## Flexor Retinaculum

It stretches between:

1. *Medially:* Pisiform bone and hamate
2. *Laterally:* Scaphoid and trapezium

## Extensor Retinaculum

Extensor retinaculum lies as a 2 cm oblique broad band sloping medially between:

1. Pisiform, triquetral and styloid process of ulna (medially) and
2. lower part of radius (laterally).

# Chapter 17 SEQs

1. Name all flexors of elbow joint and the nerves supplying them. If the nerve to chief flexors is injured in a patient, which part of his upper limb will have sensory loss?

2. a. Write anatomical features and functions of palmar aponeurosis.
   b. What is Dupuytren's contracture?

3. a. Draw and label a diagram showing the formation of cords of brachial plexus.
   b. Name the muscles supplied by long thoracic nerve and dorsal scapular nerve.

4. A five years old child was suddenly lifted by his upper limbs into the school bus. He started crying and complained of pain in his right arm. He held his elbow in flexed position with forearm pronated. In the hospital, he was treated for subluxation of head of radius.
   a. Name the joint involved and mention its type, articulating bones and ligaments.
   b. Write the cause of subluxation and its associated pain in this case.

5. a. Draw and label diagrams of clavicle to show attachments of muscles and ligaments.
   b. What is the role of these muscles and ligaments after fracture of clavicle occurs? Which is the weakest part of the clavicle?

6. A young boy fell on the ground and fractured medial epicondyle of his right arm. He did not get any treatment and later developed claw hand deformity.
   a. Which nerve has been injured in this fracture?
   b. Write the origin and course of this arm?
   c. Which muscles are responsible for his claw hand deformity?

7. a. Write the name of the nerve injured in the following clinical pictures.
   i. Winging of scapula
   ii. Wrist drop
   iii. Klumpke's paralysis
   iv. Carpal tunnel syndrome
   v. Inability to raise trunk with the upper limb during climbing

   b. List the contents of cubital fossa.

8. Name the muscles present in hypothenar compartment. Write their attachments, nerve supply and actions.

9. Write the origin, course and branches of the radial nerve. Enlist the effects of its paralysis.

10. Compare the palmar and dorsal interossei in table form.

11. Give an account of palmar spaces. What is space of parona?

12. Name the movements of the thumb. Which muscles produce these movements.

# SECTION 3

# LOWER LIMB

## CONTENTS


| | | |
|---|---|---|
| 18 | Thigh | 151 |
| 19 | Gluteal region | 165 |
| 20 | Popliteal fossa and knee | 179 |
| 21 | The leg | 191 |
| 22 | The foot | 201 |
| 23 | Miscellaneous | 215 |
| 24 | SEQs | 223 |

Chapter

# 18 THIGH

**Thigh** is the region of the lower limb lying above the knee. It is anatomically divided into three compartments:

1. Anterior or extensor compartment
2. Posterior or flexor compartment
3. Medial or adductor compartment

## FASCIA LATA

- It is the deep fascia of the thigh which invests the thighs like stockings.
- It is continuous directly with the periosteum of underlying bones or indirectly through the intermuscular septa.
- It is the continuation of the membranous layer of the superficial fascia of the abdominal wall (fascia Scarpa). It fuses with fascia Scarpa at the flexure skin crease of the hip joint.
- The upper end of fascia lata is large and has a vertical slit like cut on the front of thigh.
- The cut edges of the slit overlap to form the margins of *saphenous opening.*
- The lateral strip of the fascia lata thickens to form the *iliotibial tract.*
- The medial part of the fascia is thin and forms the cribriform fascia.
- Fascia Lata sends three intermuscular (medial, lateral and, posterior) septa to be attached on linea aspera of femur which divide the thigh into three compartments which contain:
  a. Anteriorly and laterally, the extensor group of muscles and femoral nerve,
  b. Medially, the adductor muscles and obturator nerve,
  c. Posteriorly, the flexor (Hamstrings) muscles and sciatic nerve.

## Superior Attachments of Fascia Lata at the Root of Limb

- Anteriorly to the inguinal ligament
- Laterally to the external lip of the iliac crest
- Medially to the body and inferior ramus of pubis and to the ramus and tuberosity of ischium
- Posteriorly to the sacrotuberous ligament and sacrum

## Inferior Attachments of Fascia Lata at Knee

- Anteriorly to patella
- Laterally to femoral and tibial condyles and the head of fibula
- Posteriorly to popliteal fossa
- Inferiorly to the deep fascia of the calf

Fascia lata is firmly attached with the fascia scarpa near the inguinal ligament. The line of attachment is called *Holden's line*. This line of fusion is about 8 cm long. This fusion line prevents the passage of urine into the thigh in case of damage to urethra by injury.

## Saphenous Opening

- This is a slit like oblique space lying between the cut edges of the upper part of fascia lata below the inguinal ligament.
- It is located 4 cm below and lateral to the pubic tubercle.
- The lateral margin of the slit is attached to the pubic tubercle and inguinal ligament. It forms the crescent shaped falciform margin.
- The medial cut edge is tucked deep. It passes posterior to the femoral sheath over the pectineus muscle and is attached to pectineal line of pubic bone.
- The saphenous opening is covered by loose fascia pierced by a number of structures. It is thus called as *cribriform fascia*. This fascia is pierced by:
  1. Great saphenous vein
  2. Tributaries of great saphenous vein
     a. superficial epigastric vein
     b. superficial circumflex iliac vein
     c. superficial external pudendal vein
  3. Efferent lymphatics from the superficial inguinal nodes

## Iliotibial Tract

- This is a 6 cm broad band like thickening of fascia lata on the lateral side of thigh.
- It passes vertically down.
- Upper end is attached to iliac crest.
- Lower end is attached onto the lateral condyles of the tibia.
- Lateral intermuscular septum extends from its deeper surface and is attached on the linea aspera of the femur.
- The muscles inserted into iliotibial tract are
  a. Tensor fascia lata and
  b. 3/4$^{th}$ gluteus maximus.
- It stabilizes and supports the knee joint in standing position.

## Tensor Fasciae Latae

### *Origin*

External lip of iliac crest extending from anterior superior iliac spine to iliac tubercle

### *Insertion*

Iliotibial tract

### *Nerve supply*

Superior gluteal nerve

### *Actions*

1. Extends the knee joint by pulling the iliotibial tract
2. Stabilizes the pelvis during walking

# CUTANEOUS NERVES OF THE LOWER LIMB

## Gluteal Region

1. Subcostal nerve
2. Iliohypogastric nerve
3. Posterior rami of L1, L2, L3
4. Posterior rami of S1, S2, S3

5. Lateral cutaneous nerve of thigh
6. Posterior cutaneous nerve of thigh
7. Perforating nerve of thigh

## Front and Medial Side of Thigh

1. Ilioinguinal nerve
2. Femoral branch of genitofemoral nerve
3. Lateral cutaneous nerve of thigh
4. Intermediate cutaneous nerve of thigh
5. Medial cutaneous nerve of thigh
6. Obturator nerve

## Back of Thigh

Posterior cutaneous nerve of thigh

## Front of Leg

1. Lateral cutaneous nerve of thigh
2. Superficial peroneal nerve
3. Saphenous nerve

## Back of Leg

1. Posterior cutaneous nerve of thigh
2. Lateral cutaneous nerve of calf
3. Sural nerve
4. Saphenous nerve

## Dorsum of Foot

1. Superficial peroneal nerve
2. Deep peroneal nerve
3. Saphenous nerve
4. Sural nerve

## Sole of Foot

1. Medial calcaneal nerve
2. Medial plantar nerve
3. Lateral plantar nerve

## Dermatomes

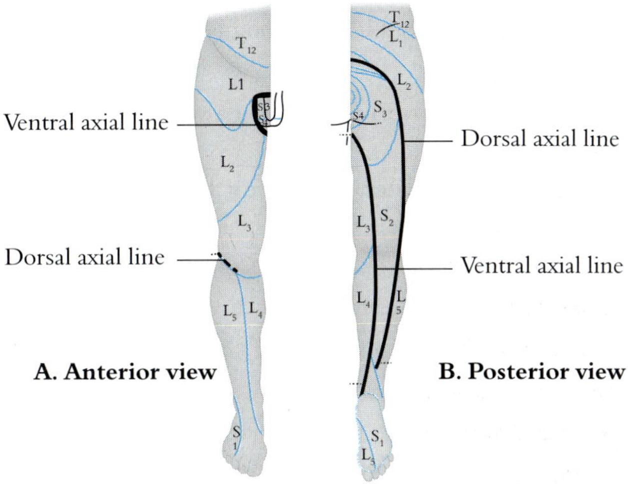


**Fig. 18.1: Dermatomes of the lower limb**

## FEMORAL TRIANGLE

It is a triangular space lying under the deep fascia on the front of thigh. The floor is gutter shaped with the apex directed downwards and leading to the adductor canal.

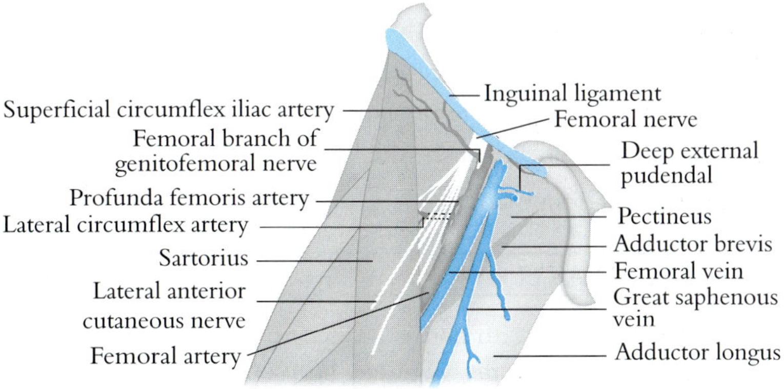


**Fig. 18.2: Boundaries and contents of femoral triangle**

### *Boundaries*

- *Lateral:* Medial border of sartorius
- *Medial:* Medial border of adductor longus
- *Base:* Inguinal ligament
- *Apex:* Continuous inferiorly with a narrow intermuscular space—the *adductor canal*
- *Floor:* (from medial to lateral) adductor longus, pectineous, psoas major, and iliacus
- *Roof:* Skin and superficial fascia. The superficial fascia contains:
  - Upper part of great saphenous vein
  - Femoral branch of genitofemoral nerve
  - Branches of ilioinguinal nerve
  - Superficial branches of femoral artery
  - Tributaries of femoral vein and
  - Superficial inguinal lymph nodes and vessels

### *Contents*

1. Femoral artery
2. Profunda femoris artery
3. Lateral circumflex artery
4. Medial circumflex artery
5. Deep external pudendal artery
6. Femoral vein and its tributaries
7. Femoral nerve
8. Femoral branch of genitofemoral nerve
9. Lateral cutaneous nerve of the thigh
10. Deep inguinal lymph nodes

## FEMORAL SHEATH

It is a funnel shaped sheath and is an extension of the fascial lining of the abdomen behind the inguinal ligament. Abdominal vessels (external iliac vein and artery) course into the thigh through this facial sheath and acquire the name of femoral vein and artery respectively.

- It surrounds the upper 4 cm of the femoral artery and vein.

- It lies behind the medial part of inguinal ligament.
- Anteriorly, it consists of fascia transversalis.
- Posteriorly, it consists of the fascia iliaca.
- Lateral to it lies the lacunar ligament.
- It is partitioned into three compartments:
  - Lateral part encloses the femoral artery and femoral branch of genitofemoral nerve.
  - Middle part encloses the femoral vein.
  - Medial part is a short space called *femoral canal.*

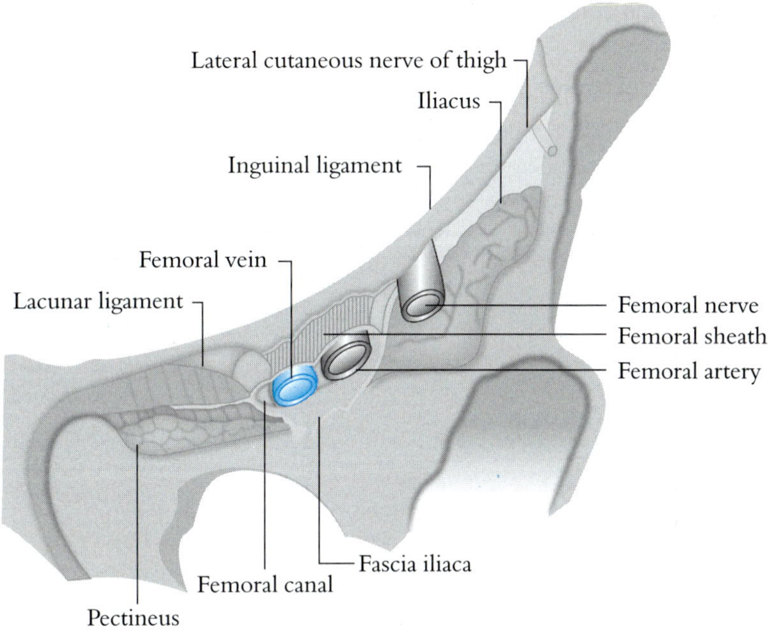


**Fig. 18.3: Femoral sheath and its content**

## Femoral Canal

- It is a short fascial tube of the medial compartment of the femoral sheath.
- The canal lies posterior to the saphenous opening and the cribriform fascia.
- The upper wide end of the canal is called as *femoral ring*. It is separated from the abdominal cavity by the peritoneum only.

- The boundaries of the femoral ring are:
  - Anteriorly, inguinal ligament,
  - Posteriorly, pectin pubis,
  - Medially, sharp edge of lacunar ligament and
  - Laterally, femoral vein.
- Lower end of the canal is closed by the fusion of its walls.
- The significance of the femoral canal is that it allows the expansion of femoral vein within the femoral sheath in case of large venous returns.
- It is also the potential site for the femoral hernia.
- The canal contains loose fatty tissue, a small lymph node and few lymph vessels.

**Table 18.1: Muscles of the Anterior Compartment of Thigh**

| Muscle | Origin | Insertion | Nerve Supply | Actions |
|---|---|---|---|---|
| Sartorius | Anterior superior iliac spine | Upper medial part of tibia | Femoral nerve | Draws the lower limb to sitting tailor's position (thighs and knees flexed, laterally rotated and abducted) |
| Iliacus | Iliac fossa | Below the lesser trochanter of femur | Femoral nerve | Powerful flexion of hip joint |
| Psoas major | Lumbar spines L1-5 | Lesser trochanter of femur | Ventral ramus L2-3 L3 | Powerful flexion of hip joint |
| Pectineus | Pectineal line of pubis | On the line from the lesser trochanter to the linea aspera | Femoral nerve | 1. Flexion of thigh 2. Adduction of thigh |

| Muscle | Origin | Insertion | Nerve Supply | Actions |
|---|---|---|---|---|
| **Quadriceps femoris** | | | | |
| 1. Rectus femoris | *Reflected head:* groove above acetabulum<br>*Straight head:* anterior superior iliac spine | Common tendon of Quadriceps femoris is attached to the base and sides of patella. | Each muscle is supplied by a separate branch of femoral nerve. | Extension of knee joint<br><br>Rectus femoris may assist in hip flexion. |
| 2. Vastus lateralis | Greater trochanter to lateral supracondylar line | | | |
| 3. Vastus medialis | Intratrochanter line, spiral line, linea aspera and medial supracondylar line | | | |
| 4. Vastus intermedius | Anterior and lateral surface of upper 2/3rds of shaft of femur | | | |

## FEMORAL ARTERY

- It is the main artery of the lower limb and is direct continuation of the external iliac artery behind the inguinal ligament.
- It enters the thigh at mid-inguinal point where it lies over the tendon of psoas major.
- In the femoral sheath, it lies medial to femoral nerve and lateral to femoral vein.
- It descends through the femoral sheath and enters the femoral triangle deep to sartorius.
- In the femoral triangle, it is covered only by the skin and fasciae.

- It leaves the femoral triangle at its apex and enters the adductor canal along with femoral vein. Here it becomes the popliteal artery.

### Superficial Branches

1. Superficial external pudendal artery
2. Superficial epigastric artery
3. Superficial circumflex iliac artery

### Deep Branches

1. Profunda femoris artery
2. Deep external pudendal artery
3. Descending genicular artery
4. Muscular arteries

> Femoral artery is the second only choice to radial artery for the placement of an arterial line.

## FEMORAL NERVE

- It is the nerve of the extensor compartment of thigh.
- It is formed from the posterior divisions of the anterior rami of the lumbar plexus (L2, 3 and 4).
- It descends in the groove between iliacus and psoas major.
- It enters the thigh behind the inguinal ligament lateral to the femoral sheath.
- It ends 2 cm below the inguinal ligament by dividing into several branches.

### *Branches*

#### *Muscular branches*

1. Nerve to pectineus
2. Nerves to sartorius (2-3 branches)
3. Nerves to rectus femoris (2 branches)
4. Nerve to vastus medialis

5. Nerve to vastus lateralis
6. Nerves to vastus intermedius (2-3 branches)

### *Articular branches*

1. To the hip joint
2. To the knee joint

### *Cutaneous branches*

1. Saphenous nerve
2. Intermediate femoral cutaneous nerve
3. Medial femoral cutaneous nerve

## FEMORAL VEIN

- This is the direct continuation of the popliteal artery. It contains 4-5 valves.
- It begins at the opening in the adductor magnus and courses upwards in the femoral triangle to the inguinal ligament on the medial side of the femoral artery.
- Behind the mid-inguinal point, it becomes the external iliac vein.

### Tributaries

1. Corresponding vein of profunda femoris artery
2. Great saphenous vein

**Table 18.2: Muscles of the Medial Compartment of Thigh**

| Muscle | Origin | Insertion | Nerve Supply | Actions |
|---|---|---|---|---|
| Gracilis | 1. Inferior ramus of pubic bone<br>2. Body of pubis (lower half) | Medial surface of tibial shaft | Obturator nerve, anterior division | 1. Thigh adduction<br>2. Knee flexion<br>3. Medial rotation of the leg |

| Muscle | Origin | Insertion | Nerve Supply | Actions |
|---|---|---|---|---|
| Adductor longus | 1. Body of pubis<br>2. Angle between pubic crest and symphysis | Middle third of linea aspera | Obturator nerve, anterior division | 1. Adduction of thigh<br>2. Stabilizes the hip bone on femur and prevents lateral tilting of limb on walking |
| Adductor brevis | 1. Body of pubis<br>2. Inferior ramus of pubis | Upper part of linea aspera | Obturator nerve, anterior division | 1. Adduction of thigh<br>2. Stabilizes the hip bone on femur and prevents lateral tilting of limb on walking |
| Adductor magnus | *Hamstring part:* Ischial tuberosity<br>*Adductor part:* ischiopubic ramus | Medial supracondylar line, linea aspera, upto gluteal tuberosiy | 1. Hamstring part by tibial part of sciatic nerve<br>2. Adductor part by posterior division of obturator nerve | 1. Adduction of thigh<br>2. Stabilizes the hip bone on femur and prevents lateral tilting of limb on walking |
| Obturator externus | 1. Obturator membrane<br>2. Obturator foramen except its notch | Trochanteric fossa | Posterior division of obturator nerve | 1. Lateral rotation of the femur<br>2. Stabilizes and supports the pelvis |

## ADDUCTOR (HUNTER'S OR SUBSARTORIAL) CANAL

It is a deep furrow on the medial side of the thigh.

- It extends between the apex of femoral triangle to the hiatus of adductor magnus.
- The furrow lies between the vastus medialis laterally and adductor longus and magnus posteriorly.
- *Roof* is formed by a fascial layer over which stretches the Sartorius muscle, which converts it into a canal.
- Inferiorly, this fascial sheath is fused with the tendon of adductor magnus.
- There is an aperture in the tendon of adductor magnus called *adductor opening* through which femoral vessels pass into the popliteal fossa.

### *Contents*

1. Femoral artery
2. Femoral vein
3. Saphenous nerve
4. Nerve to vastus medialis
5. Terminal part of obturator nerve

## CLINICAL AND APPLIED INTEGRATION

### Femoral Hernia

The protrusion of abdominal contents into the thigh through the femoral canal is called *femoral hernia*. In standing posture, the abdominal contents press on the femoral ring which is a weak point. If there is weakening of abdominal muscles with raised intra-abdominal pressure e.g. by coughing, straining, childbirth or weight lifting etc., some part of abdominal viscera protrude through the femoral canal into the front of thigh. Commonly, a loop of small intestine is the herniated viscera. If the blood supply of the herniated loop is occluded at the sharp edge of femoral ring, the hernia becomes strangulated. It is intensely painful and if constriction at the femoral ring is not relieved urgently, gangrene of the herniated loops may start. The pressure at the neck of hernia may be relieved by surgically dividing the *lacunar ligament* forming the medial boundary of the femoral ring. This procedure will immediately restore the blood supply of the hernial sac. The hernia is surgically treated by a procedure called '*Herniorrhaphy*.' In this procedure, the contents of hernia are retracted into the abdomen and surgical repair and strengthening of abdominal wall is done by placing a special type of prolene mesh.

## Femoral Artery Catheterization

At the mid-inguinal point, femoral artery lies on the tendon of psoas major. Psoas separates it from the capsule of hip joint (and the head of femur). This is the point where *femoral pulse* can be felt. This is also the site commonly used for arterial catheterization. Its superficial position below the inguinal ligament makes it easily accessible.

A long catheter is inserted into the femoral artery under fluoroscopic guidance along the external and common iliac arteries into the aorta. The catheter may be guided in the left ventricle to obtain the pressure of the heart chambers and sometimes to introduce pace maker. Other arteries like superior and inferior mesenteric, celiac or renal arteries can also be viewed. A dye or contrast medium may be injected in the artery of interest to obtain radiograph for permanent record.

Chapter

# 19 GLUTEAL REGION

**GLUTEAL** region, commonly known as buttocks, lies behind the pelvis and above the posterior compartment of thigh. It extends from the iliac crest to the gluteal folds.

**Table 19.1: Muscles of the Gluteal Region**

| Muscle | Origin | Insertion | Nerve Supply | Actions |
|---|---|---|---|---|
| Gluteus maximus | 1. Ilium (external surface) behind posterior gluteal line<br>2. Back of sacrum and coccyx<br>3. Sacrotuberous ligament | 1. ¼ into gluteal tuberosity<br>2. ¾ into iliotibial tract | Inferior gluteal nerve | 1. Extension of the hip joint chiefly in running, climbing stairs and lifting heavy weight<br>2. Lateral rotation of hip joint<br>3. Extension of knee through iliotibial tract<br>4. The chief antigravity muscle during the act of sitting |
| Gluteus medius | Anterior and posterior gluteal lines of ilium | Greater trochanter | Superior gluteal nerve | 1. When the limb is free to move, these muscles abduct the thigh. |

| Muscle | Origin | Insertion | Nerve Supply | Actions |
|---|---|---|---|---|
| Gluteus minimus | Anterior and posterior gluteal lines of ilium | Greater trochanter | Superior gluteal nerve | 2. When the limb is supporting body weight, they tilt the pelvis so that the opposite foot can be raised from the ground.<br>3. Medial rotation of thigh by anterior fibers |
| Piriformis | Pelvic surface of S2, S3, S4 | Upper border of greater trochanter | S1, S2 | *Acting as prime movers:*<br>1. Lateral rotators of the extended thigh<br>2. Abduction of the flexed thigh<br>*Acting together:*<br>Adjust and stabilize the hip joint. Maintain the head of femur in the acetabulum |
| Obturator internus | Pelvic surface of obturator membrane | Medial surface of greater trochanter | L5; S1, S2 | |
| Gemellus superior | Superior margin of lesser sciatic notch | Tendon of obturator internus | Nerve to obturator internus | |
| Gemellus inferior | Ischial tuberosity, inferior margin of lesser sciatic notch | Tendon of obturator interus | Nerve to quadratus femoris | |
| Quadratus femoris | Lateral margin of ischial tuberosity | Back of greater trochanter | Nerve to quadratus femoris (L4-5; S1) | |

## STRUCTURES LYING DEEP TO GLUTEUS MAXIMUS

### Muscles

1. Gluteus medius
2. Gluteus minimus
3. Reflected head of rectus femoris
4. Obturator internus
5. Obturator externus
6. Gemelli (superior and inferior)
7. Hamstrings origin

### Nerves

1. Sciatic nerve
2. Superior gluteal nerve
3. Inferior gluteal nerve
4. Pudendal nerve
5. Posterior cutaneous nerve of thigh
6. Nerve to quadratus femoris
7. Nerve to obturator internus

### Blood Vessels

1. Superior gluteal artery and vein
2. Inferior gluteal artery and vein
3. Internal pudendal artery and vein
4. Ascending branch of medial femoral circumflex artery

### Anastomoses

1. Trochanteric anastomosis
2. Cruciate anastomosis

### Joints and Ligaments

1. Sacroiliac and hip joints
2. Sacrotuberous ligament
3. Sacrospinous ligament
4. Ischiofemoral ligament

## Bursae

1. Bursa over greater trochanter
2. Bursa over ischial tuberosity
3. Bursa over vastus lateralis

## Foramina of Gluteal Region

### *Greater sciatic foramen*

- It is formed by the greater sciatic notch, sacrotuberous and sacrospinous ligaments.
- It provides a passage from the pelvis into the gluteal region.

### *Structures passing through the foramen*

Muscle:

1. Piriformis

Nerves:

2. Sciatic nerve
3. Posterior cutaneous nerve of thigh
4. Superior gluteal nerve
5. Inferior gluteal nerve
6. Pudendal nerve
7. Nerve to obturator internus and quadratus femoris

Vessels:

8. Superior gluteal artery and vein
9. Inferior gluteal artery and vein
10. Internal pudendal artery and vein

### *Lesser sciatic foramen*

- It is formed by the lesser sciatic notch, sacrotuberous and sacrospinous ligaments.
- It provides an entrance to the structures of gluteal region to the perineum.

### *Structures passing through the foramen*

Muscle:

1. Tendon of obturator internus

Nerves:

2. Pudendal nerve
3. Nerve to obturator internus

Vessels:

4. Internal pudendal artery and vein

## Trochanteric Anastomosis

- It is located near the trochanteric fossa.
- Main source of blood supply to head of femur
- Anastomosis is formed by:
  1. The descending branch of superior gluteal artery,
  2. The ascending branch of medial circumflex femoral artery,
  3. The ascending branch of lateral circumflex femoral artery,
  4. The inferior gluteal artery and
  5. The first perforating branch of profunda femoris artery.
- Branches from the anastomosis course with the *retinacular fibers* of the capsule along the neck of femur to supply its head.
- It is a connection between the internal iliac artery and the femoral artery.

> Intracapsular fracture of the neck of femur leads to the rupture of retinacular fibers of the capsule and contained vessels. It usually causes *avascular necrosis of the head of femur*.

## Cruciate Anastomosis

- It is located at the level of the lower border of the middle of lesser trochanter.
- The anastomosing arteries are:
  1. Transverse branch of medial circumflex femoral artery,
  2. Transverse branch of lateral circumflex femoral artery,
  3. Ascending branch of first perforating artery,
  4. Descending branch of inferior gluteal artery.
- It is a connection between the internal iliac and femoral artery.

**Table 19.2: Muscles of the Posterior Compartment (Hamstring) of Thigh**

| Muscle | Origin | Insertion | Nerve Supply | Actions |
|---|---|---|---|---|
| Biceps femoris | *Long head:* ischial tuberosity<br>*Short head:* linea aspera, lateral supracon-dylar ridge | Head of fibula | *Long head:* tibial nerve<br>*Short head:* common peroneal nerve | 1. Flexor of knee joint<br>2. Lateral rotator of leg<br>3. Long head: extensor of hip joint |
| Semiten-dinosis | Ischial tuberosity | Upper part medial surface of shaft of tibia | Tibial nerve | 1. Flexor of knee joint<br>2. Medial rotator of leg<br>3. Extensor of hip joint |
| Semimem-branous | Ischial tuberosity | Medial of condyle of tibia | Tibial nerve | 1. Flexor of knee joint<br>2. Medial rotator of leg<br>3. Extensor of hip joint |
| Adductor magnus (hamstring part) | Ischial tuberosity | Adductor tubercle of femur | Tibial nerve | Extensor of hip joint |

## LUMBAR PLEXUS

### *Origin*

Ventral rami of upper four lumbar nerves i.e. L1, 2, 3 and L4

## Location

It is formed in the substance of psoas major.

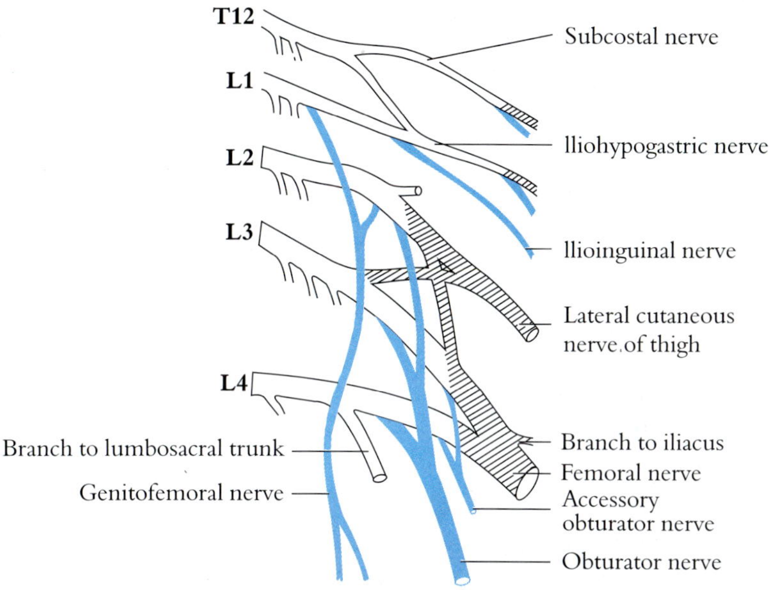


**Fig. 19.1: Formation of lumbar plexus and its branches**

## Branches

### From anterior division

1. Iliohypogastric nerve (L1)
2. Ilioinguinal (L1)
3. Genitofemoral (L1, 2)
4. Obturator nerve ( L2, 3, 4)

### From posterior division

1. Lateral femoral cutaneous nerve (L2, 3)
2. Femoral nerve (L2, 3, 4)
3. Nerve to lumbosacral trunk (L4, 5)

# SACRAL PLEXUS

## *Origin*

It is formed by the lumbosacral trunk (L4, 5) and the anterior rami of upper four sacral nerves (S1, 2, 3, 4).

## *Location*

It is formed in front of piriformis muscle in the pelvis.

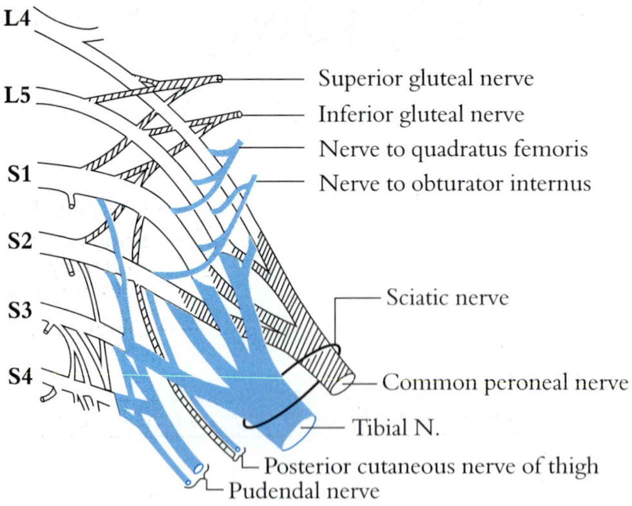


**Fig. 19.2: Sacral plexus and its branches**

## *Branches*

### *From the cord*

1. Posterior cutaneous nerve (S1, 2, 3)
2. Nerve to piriformis (S1, 2)
3. Perforating cutaneous nerve (S2, 3)
4. Pudendal nerve (S2, 3, 4)
5. Pelvic splanchnic nerves (S2, 3, 4)

### *From ventral division*

1. Tibial nerve (L4, 5; S1, 2, 3)

2. Nerve to quadratus femoris and inferior gemellus (L4, 5; S1)
3. Nerve to obturator internus and superior gemellus (L4, 5; S1)

### *From the dorsal division*

1. Common peroneal nerve (L4, 5; S1, 2, 3)
2. Superior gluteal nerve (L4, 5; S1)
3. Inferior gluteal nerve (L5, S1, 2)

## Sciatic Nerve

- This is the thickest nerve of the body.
- It arises from the sacral plexus in the pelvis from spinal roots L4-5; S1-3.
- It passes from the great sciatic foramen into the gluteal region deep to gluteus maximus.
- It courses vertically through the hamstring compartment deep to the long head of biceps. Here it lies between biceps and adductor magnus.
- At the apex of popliteal fossa, it divides into its tibial and common peroneal components.

### *Branches*

1. Common peroneal nerve
2. Tibial nerve
3. Muscular—nerves to hamstring muscles
4. Articular—to the hip joint

Compression of the sciatic nerve against the femur, as sometimes happens after sitting for a long time on hard surface, leads to temporary sensory disturbance along its area of cutaneous distribution called *paresthesia*. One of the clinical conditions resulting from the compression of this nerve is known as '*sleeping foot*'. The condition reverses after the compression is released.

# HIP JOINT

## Type

It is a multiaxial synovial joint of ball and socket variety.

## Articulating Bones

1. Head of the femur
2. Acetabulum formed by the fusion:
   a. Ilium
   b. Ischium
   c. Pubis

## Capsule

- The capsule is loose but extremely strong.
- Capsule is attached circumferentially around the labrum and transverse ligament.
- Laterally, it extends to the neck of femur to be attached.
- In front, it is attached to the intertrochanteric line.
- At the back, it is attached in the middle of femoral neck.
- From the attachments of capsule, *retinacular fibers* reflect back to the articular margin of femur. Nutrient arteries pass through these fibers to supply the head of femur.

## Ligaments

These are three in number and arise from one of the each constituent bone of hip joint.

1. Iliofemoral ligament is the strongest of all and arises from ilium.
2. Pubofemoral arises from superior ramus of pubic bone.
3. Ischiopubic arises from the ischium.

## Blood Supply

1. Medial circumflex femoral artery
2. Obturator artery in the ligament of head of femur

## Nerve Supply

1. Femoral nerve via nerve to rectus femoris
2. Obturator nerve
3. Sciatic nerve

The femoral, obturator and sciatic nerves also supply the knee joint. The pain arising in the hip joint may be referred to the knee joint.

## Movements

*Flexion (range: 120°)*

1. Psoas major
2. Iliacus

Assisted by:

3. Rectus femoris, sartorius and pectineus

*Extension (20°)*

1. Gluteus maximus
2. Hamstrings

*Abduction (60°)*

1. Gluteus medius
2. Gluteus minimus

Assisted by:

3. Tensor fascia lata and sartorius

*Adduction (30°)*

1. Pectineus
2. Adductors (longus, brevis, and magnus)
3. Gracilis

*Medial rotation (40°)*

1. Gluteus medius
2. Gluteus minimus

Assisted by:

3. Tensor fascia lata

*Lateral rotation (40°)*

1. Piriformis
2. Obturator internus and externus
3. Superior and inferior gemelli
4. Quadratus femoris

Assisted by:

5. Gluteus maximus and sartorius

*Circumduction:* It is a combination of all the movements.

## Factors Stabilizing the Hip Joint

### 1. *Bony factors*

a. Adaptation of acetabulum and femoral head to each other
b. Length and obliquity of neck of femur

### 2. *Ligaments*

a. Iliofemoral
b. Ischiofemoral
c. Pubofemoral

### 3. *Muscles*

Small muscles of the gluteal region i.e. piriformis, obturator internus and externus, gemelli, quadratus femoris

### 4. *Glenoid labrum*

Deepening of the joint cavity by the glenoid labrum

### 5. *Posture*

The joint is less stable when it is flexed and adducted.

### 6. *Others*

Atmospheric pressure

## CLINICAL AND APPLIED INTEGRATION

### Gluteal Intramuscular Injection

Gluteal region extends from the iliac crest to the gluteal fold. The upper outer quadrant is a common site for intramuscular injections especially in children. It is the safe region to avoid damage to the sciatic nerve.

### Congenital Dislocation of Hip Joint

Congenital dislocation of hip joint is a common occurrence in which femoral head is not located in the acetabulum. More than 50% cases are bilateral and girls are affected eight times more than boys. Affected limb is shorter and there is inability to abduct the thigh. Trendelenburg's sign is also positive in these cases.

## Coxa Vara And Valga

The angle of inclination i.e. angle between the neck of femur and femoral shaft is 1200-1300 in adults. It varies with age and sex. In children, it is 1600. The angle of inclination decreases in *coxa vara* and can be seen in fracture of neck of femur. In *coxa valga* this angle is more than the normal angle. Coxa valga occurs in cases of congenital dislocation of the hip. *Shenton's line,* which is a curved line between the inferior margin of the neck of femur and superior margin of the obturator foramen, is disrupted in both of these conditions.

## Sciatica

It is defined as the shooting pain along the distribution of the sciatic nerve. It is caused by compression or irritation of one or more roots of the sciatic nerve. The most common cause is prolapse of one or more of the vertebral discs spontaneously or as a result of injury.

## Waddling Gait (Lurching Gait)

It occurs due to the unilateral paralysis of the gluteus medius and gluteus minimus muscles. Patient usually sways towards the paralysed side in an attempt to clear the opposite foot off the ground. When the patient stands on one leg with the opposite foot off the ground, pelvis on the unsupported side sinks (positive *Trendelenburg test*).

In case of *paralysis of gluteus maximus*, the patient cannot rise from the sitting position. He/she typically stands up with support placing hands first on the legs and then on the thighs.

Chapter

# 20 POPLITEAL FOSSA AND KNEE

**POPLITEAL FOSSA** is a diamond shaped space behind the knee.

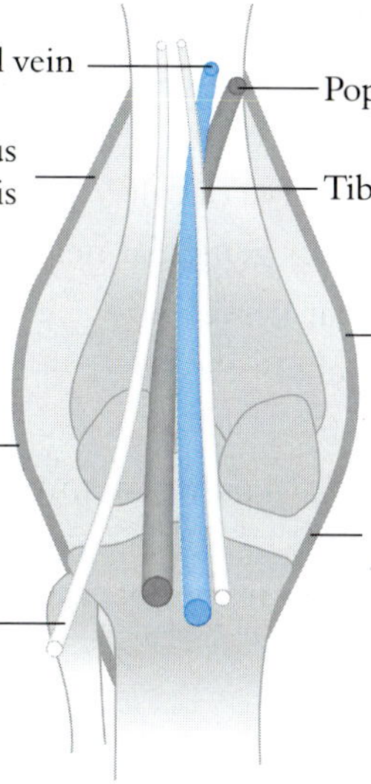


**Fig. 20.1: Boundaries and contents of popliteal fossa**

## Boundaries

**Superomedial:** Semimembranous and semitendinosus

**Superolateral:** Biceps femoris

**Inferomedal:** Medial head of gastrocnemius

**Inferolateral:** Lateral head of gastrocnemius and plantaris

**Roof:** Skin, fascia lata

**Floor** is formed from above downwards by:

1. Femur,
2. Capsule of knee joint,
3. Oblique popliteal ligament and
4. Popliteal muscle.

## Contents

1. Popliteal artery and its branches:
   a. Muscular branches and sural arteries (two) supplying two heads of gastrocnemius
   b. Superior and inferior medial genicular arteries
   c. Superior and inferior lateral genicular arteries
   d. Middle genicular artery
2. Popliteal vein and its branches (same as that of popliteal artery)
3. Small saphenous vein which drains into popliteal vein
4. Common peroneal nerve and its branches:
   a. Sural communicating nerve
   b. Lateral cutaneous nerve of calf
   c. Superior and inferior genicular nerves
   d. Recurrent genicular nerve
5. Tibial nerve and branches:
   a. Sural nerve
   b. Muscular branches to gastrocnemius, plantaris, popliteus and soleus
   c. Genicular branches (superior medial, inferior medial and middle)
6. Popliteal lymph nodes
7. Connective tissue and pad of fat

## POPLITEAL ARTERY

### Origin

It is the continuation of femoral artery. It starts from the hiatus in the adductor magnus.

### Termination

It ends at the fibrous arch of the soleus muscle.

### Relations

- It lies deep and medial to the sciatic nerve and tibial nerve in the upper part of the fossa.
- In the middle part, it lies lateral to the tibial nerve.

- Below the fibrous arch of soleus, it again returns to the medial side of the artery.
- Popliteal vein remains in between the nerve and artery throughout its course in the fossa.

### *Branches*

1. Medial superior genicular artery
2. Medial inferior genicular artery
3. Lateral superior genicular artery
4. Lateral inferior genicular artery
5. Middle genicular artery
6. Two sural arteries supplying two heads of gastrocnemius
7. Other muscular branches

Popliteal artery pulsation can be can be felt at the back of the popliteal fossa against the back of the femur when the knee is slightly flexed.

## ANASTOMOSIS AROUND KNEE JOINT

The following arteries participate in the anastomosis around the knee joint:

Branches of **Popliteal Artery:**

1. Medial superior genicular artery
2. Medial inferior genicular artery
3. Lateral superior genicular artery
4. Lateral inferior genicular artery
5. Middle genicular artery

Branches of **Femoral Artery:**

1. Descending genicular branch

Branches of **Lateral Circumflex Femoral Artery:**

1. Descending branch

Branches of **Anterior Tibial Artery:**

1. Anterior recurrent artery
2. Posterior recurrent artery

Branches of **Posterior Tibial Artery:**

1. Circumflex fibular branch

## POPLITEAL VEIN

### *Origin*

It is formed by the union of the anterior and posterior tibial veins and their venae comitantes.

### *Termination*

It continues as femoral vein at the hiatus of adductor magnus.

### *Relations*

Throughout its course, it lies between the popliteal artery and tibial nerve.

### *Tributaries*

1. Branches corresponding to the branches of femoral artery
2. Small saphenous vein

## POPLITEUS

### *Origin*

It originates from a triangular area above the soleal line on the back of tibia.

### *Insertion*

The tendon of the muscle is intracapsular within the cavity of the knee joint. It inserts into the:

1. Groove on the lateral surface of the lateral condyle of femur,
2. Arcuate popliteal ligament,
3. Posterior convexity of the lateral meniscus and
4. Capsule of knee joint.

### *Nerve supply*

Tibial nerve

### *Action*

1. In the erect position, it *laterally rotates* the femur at the commencement of flexion to unlock the knee.

2. In the fully extended knee, fermur rotates medially on the tibia to lock the knee joint.
3. In the sitting position, it *medially rotates* the tibia at the commencement of flexion.

## TIBIAL NERVE

### Origin

It begins at the apex of popliteal fossa, as a separate component of sciatic nerve.

### Course

- From the apex of popliteal fossa, it descends vertically in the middle of the fossa.
- It passes deep to the heads of gastrocnemius.
- It passes under the fibrous arch of the soleus.
- Below the arch, it enters the calf.

### Branches

#### *Motor branches*

1. Plantaris
2. Gastrocnemius
3. Soleus
4. Popliteus

#### *Articular branches*

1. Superior medial genicular branch
2. Inferior medial genicular branch
3. Middle genicular branch

#### *Cutaneous branch*

1. Sural nerve

#### *Terminal branches*

1. Medial plantar nerve
2. Lateral plantar nerve

## COMMON PERONEAL (FIBULAR) NERVE

### *Origin*

It begins at the apex of popliteal fossa as a separate component of sciatic nerve.

### *Course*

- Descends downward and laterally
- Remains medial to the biceps tendon
- Pierces through the substance of peroneus longus to lie at the neck of fibula

### *Termination*

It ends in the substance of peroneus longus by dividing into its terminal branches.

### *Branches*

1. Sural communicating nerve
2. Lateral cutaneous nerve of the calf
3. Superior genicular nerve
4. Inferior genicular nerve
5. Recurrent genicular nerve
6. Muscular branches to short head of biceps femoris
7. Superficial peroneal nerve (terminal branch)
8. Deep peroneal nerve (terminal branch)

> At the neck of the fibula, this nerve can be felt in living persons by rolling it against the neck.

## KNEE JOINT

It is a synovial joint of modified hinge variety. It is the largest joint of the body. It is a compound joint comprising of :

1. **Two condylar joints** between the medial and lateral condyles of femur and the corresponding condyles of tibia
2. **Sellar (saddle) joint** between the patella and the femur

## Articulating Structures

1. Medial and lateral condyles of the femur
2. Medial and lateral plateaus (corresponding articular surfaces) of the tibia
3. Patella

> Keep in mind that fibula is not directly involved in the articulation of knee joint.

## Menisci

1. Medial meniscus
2. Lateral meniscus

## Ligaments

### *1. Extracapsular ligaments*

a. Ligamentum Patellae, is a continuation of the quadriceps femoris tendon attached superiorly to the lower border of patella and inferiorly to the tibial tuberosity. In fact, it is the most powerful factor which stabilizes the knee joint.

b. Lateral collateral ligament

c. Medial collateral ligament

d. Oblique popliteal ligament

### *2. Intracapsular ligaments*

a. Anterior cruciate ligament

b. Posterior cruciate ligament

c. Anterior and posterior meniscofemoral ligaments

d. Transverse ligament

e. Arcuate popliteal ligament

> The *posterior cruciate ligaments* prevent posterior displacement of the tibia on the femur when one walks downstairs or downhill.

## Capsule of Knee Joint

### *Superior attachment of capsule*

- Posteriorly to the upper margins of the medial and lateral condyles of femur and intercondylar fossa
- Medially to the articular margin of the femur
- Laterally proximal to the popliteus tendon groove on the femur
- Anteriorly blends with the patellar retinacula but is deficient above the patella

### *Inferior attachment of capsule*

- Posteriorly to the margins of tibial condyles and intercondylar area
- Medially to the margins of tibial condyles except by the passage for the tendon of popliteus tendon on the lateral condyle
- Laterally to the head of the fibula
- Anteriorly from the capsule is fused with the sides of tibial condyles and patellar retinacula to the tibial tuberosity

## Synovial Membrane

It is attached to the articular margins of the femur, tibia and patella. It lines the internal surface of the capsule. It is separated from the capsule by the popliteus tendon and cruciate ligaments which lie outside the synovial cavity.

## Bursae

### *Anterior bursae*

1. Suprapatellar bursa
2. Prepatellar bursa
3. Superficial infrapatellar bursa
4. Deep infrapatellar bursa

### *Posterior bursae*

1. Popliteal bursa
2. Semimembranous bursa
3. Four bursae are related to the tendons of insertion of biceps femoris, sartorius, gracilis and semitendinosus muscles.

## Nerve Supply

Articular branches from:

1. Femoral nerve
2. Obturator nerve
3. Common peroneal nerve
4. Tibial nerve

## Blood Supply

1. Capsule and joint are supplied by the five genicular arteries.
2. Cruciate ligaments are supplied by the middle genicular artery.

## Factors Stabilizing the Knee Joint

1. Bony configuration and intercondylar eminence of the tibia
2. Ligaments
3. Muscles
4. Menisci

## Movements at the Knee Joint

### *Flexion*

1. Biceps femoris
2. Semimembranous
3. Semitendinosus

Assisted by:

4. Gracilis, sartorius, popliteus, gastrocnemius and plantaris

### *Extension*

1. Quadriceps femoris

Assisted by:

2. Tensor fasciae latae

### *Lateral rotation*

1. Biceps femoris

### *Medial rotation*

1. Semimembranous
2. Semitendinosus

Flexion and extension take place in the upper compartment of knee joint above the menisci. The medial and lateral rotations take place below the menisci in the lower compartment of the joint.

### *Mechanism of locking and unlocking of the knee*

At the end of extension of knee joint, tibia slightly rotates medially to lock the knee joint. However, to unlock the joint, popliteus laterally rotates the tibia as the flexion starts.

## CLINICAL AND APPLIED INTEGRATION

### Guy Ropes and Bursa Ansarina

A group of three muscles sharing one muscle from each compartment of the thigh and having common insertion on the medial subcutaneous surface of the shaft of tibia, is called as guy ropes. These muscles descend in the following order:

1. Sartorius of anterior compartment of thigh converges from the ilium supplied by femoral nerve.
2. Gracilis of medial compartment of thigh converges from the pubic bone supplied by obturator nerve.
3. Semitendinosus of posterior compartment of thigh converges from the ischium supplied by sciatic nerve.

These muscles stabilize the bony pelvis on the femur by holding and supporting each constituent part of the hip bone by a separate muscle of its own compartment.

***Bursa Ansarina*** separates the tendons of guy rope muscles from each other at their insertion and also from the tibial collateral ligament.

### Genu Valgum (Knock Knee)

The angle between the long axis of thigh and the leg (called as Q-angle) is larger than normal. The leg is abnormally abducted called as genu valgum or knock knee.

### Genu Varum (Bow Knee)

The angle between the long axis of thigh and leg (i.e. Q-angle) is abnormally small. This condition is known as genu varum deformity of the knee.

## Housemaid's Knee

This condition is caused by prepatellar bursitis due to repeated trauma of this bursa leading to the enlargement of prepatellar bursa. It occurs in those housemaids who scrub the floor on their hands and knee in the kneeling position.

## Miner's Knee

This condition usually occurs in coal miners. Repeated friction of prepatellar bursa leads to the infection of the prepatellar bursa called miner's knee.

## Hamstring Injuries

Hamstring injuries i.e. pulled or torn muscles commonly occur in athletes and players who take part in quick start sports. Individuals participating in running, jumping, football, hockey and basketball are more prone to hamstring injuries.

## Baker's Cyst

It is the protrusion of synovial membrane through a hole located in the center of the posterior part of the capsule of knee joint. It results due to osteoarthritis.

## Common Peroneal Nerve Injury

This nerve is very vulnerable to injury due to:

1. Exposure to direct trauma at the neck of fibula and
2. Fracture of upper end of fibula.

The lesion of common peroneal nerve leads to:

1. Foot drop,
2. Sensory loss over the lateral side of the back of the leg and
3. Sensory loss over the dorsum of the foot and toes.

Chapter

# 21 THE LEG

**THE LEG** is the region of lower limb which extends from the knee to the ankle. It consists of three fascial compartments. The muscles of the three compartments are covered by the deep fascia of the leg. Two intermuscular septae from its deep surface of the fascia pass inwards to become attached on the fibula. The compartments of the leg are:

1. Anterior compartment lies between the anterior intermuscular septum and tibia.
2. Posterior compartment lies between the posterior intermuscular septum and the tibia. This compartment is also called calf of the leg. The muscles in this compartment are divided into two groups i.e. superficial and deep by the *Transverse fascia*. Superficial group conists of gastrocnemius, plantaris and soleus muscles whereas deep group contains flexor digitorum longus, flexor hallucis longus and tibialis posterior.
3. Lateral compartment lies on the fibular side between the anterior and posterior intermuscular septae.

**Table 21.1: Muscles of the Anterior (Extensor) Compartment of Leg**

| Muscle | Origin | Insertion | Nerve Supply | Actions |
|---|---|---|---|---|
| Tibialis Anterior | 1. Upper 2/3rd of extensor surface of tibia<br>2. Interosseous membrane | 1. Medial and inferior surfaces of medial cuneiform<br>2. 1st metatarsal | Deep peroneal nerve | 1. Dorsiflexion of ankle<br>2. Inversion of foot<br>3. Maintains medial longitudinal arch of foot |

| Muscle | Origin | Insertion | Nerve Supply | Actions |
|---|---|---|---|---|
| Extensor hallucis longus | 1. Middle half of fibula<br>2. Interosseous membrane | Base of the terminal phalanx of big toe | Deep peroneal nerve | 1. Dorsiflexion of big toe<br>2. Dorsiflexion of ankle |
| Extensor digit-orum longus | 1. Upper 3/4th of extensor surface of the fibula<br>2. Interosseous membrane | Divides into four tendons, inserted into the lateral four toes | Deep peroneal nerve | Dorsiflexion of lateral four toes |
| Peronius tertius | Lower 1/3rd of fibula | Dorsum of the base of 5th metatarsal bone | Deep peroneal nerve | 1. Eversion of foot<br>2. Dorsiflexion of foot |

**Table 21.2: Muscles of the Posterior (Flexor) Compartment of Leg**

| Muscle | Origin | Insertion | Nerve Supply | Actions |
|---|---|---|---|---|
| Gastro-cnemius | 1. Lateral head: lateral surface of lateral femoral condyle<br>2. Medial head: back of medial condyle and shaft of femur | Two heads form a dense aponeurosis which blends with the soleus aponeurosis to form tendo-calcaneus. It then inserts on middle 1/3rd of the back of calcaneus. | Tibial nerve | 1. The chief and rapid plantarflexor of the foot<br>2. Flexion of knee |

| Muscle | Origin | Insertion | Nerve Supply | Actions |
|---|---|---|---|---|
| Plantaris | Lower part of Supra-condylar line of the femur | Fuses with the medial border of tendocalcaneus | Tibial nerve | Weak plantarflexion |
| Soleus | Upper ¼$^{th}$ of the back of fibula and its head | The aponeurosis merges into tendocalcaneous to be inserted at the back of the calcaneus. | Tibial nerve | 1. Slow plantarflexion of the foot<br>2. Maintains balance in standing with extensors of the leg |
| Flexor digitorum longus | Back of tibia below soleal line | 1. In the sole of foot, it divides into four tendons which receive the insertion of flexor accessories.<br>2. Base of distal four phalanges (of 2-5 toes) | Tibial nerve | 1. Plantarflexion of lateral four toes<br>2. Plantarflexion of knee<br>3. Assists in maintaining the lateral and medial longitudinal arches |
| Flexor hallucis longus | 1. Flexor surface of fibula<br>2. Interosseous membrane | Base of the distal phalanx of big toe | Tibial nerve | 1. Flexion of the big toe<br>2. Plantarflexion of knee<br>3. Maintenance of medial longitudinal arch |

| Muscle | Origin | Insertion | Nerve Supply | Actions |
|---|---|---|---|---|
| Tibialis posterior | 1. Adjoining surfaces of tibia and fibula<br>2. Interosseous membrane | 1. Tuberosity of the navicular bone<br>2. All three cuneiform<br>3. 2nd, 3rd and 4th metatarsals | Tibial nerve | 1. Inversion of foot<br>2. Adduction of foot<br>3. Plantarflexion of ankle<br>4. Maintains medial longitudinal arch of foot |

**Table 21.3: Muscles of the Lateral (Peroneal) Compartment of Leg**

| Muscle | Origin | Insertion | Nerve Supply | Actions |
|---|---|---|---|---|
| Peroneus longus | 1. Head of fibula<br>2. Upper 2/3rd of lateral surface of fibula | 1. Base of 1st metatarsal<br>2. Medial cuneiform | Superficial peroneal nerve | 1. Eversion of the foot<br>2. Weak plantarflexion<br>3. Maintains lateral and transverse arches of foot |
| Peroneus brevis | 1. Lower 2/3rd of fibula | Tubercle at the base of 5th metatarsal bone | Superficial peroneal nerve | 1. Eversion of foot<br>2. Weak plantarflexion of foot |

## Interosseous Membrane

It is a tough membrane which extends from the interosseous border of tibia to that of fibula. The direction of the fibers is from the tibia sloping down towards the fibula i.e. inferolaterally. In the lower part, the fibers of interosseous membrane merge with the interosseous tibiofibular ligaments. It joins the fibula and tibia together and also gives attachment to the neighboring muscles. Two openings are present in the membrane.

1. A large opening in the upper part to admit the anterior tibial artery and accompanying veins to enter in the anterior compartment of the leg
2. A small opening in the lower part through which perforating branch of peroneal artery enters in the anterior fascial compartment of the leg

## ANTERIOR TIBIAL ARTERY

- It is one of the terminal branches formed at the bifurcation of popliteal artery in the calf.
- Near the fibular neck, it pierces the upper part of interosseous membrane to come forwards.
- From here, it descends vertically down on the interosseous membrane.
- It is accompanied by anterior tibial veins, one on either of the artery (venae comitantes) during its course. These veins anastomose at various intervals by cross channels.
- It crosses the tibia in front of ankle, midway between the medial and lateral malleoli below the extensor retinaculum.
- From this point, it continues its course in the dorsum of the foot as dorsalis paedis artery.

### *Branches*

1. Anterior recurrent artery
2. Posterior recurrent artery
3. Muscular branches to muscles of extensor compartment
4. Malleolar branches to malleolar regions

## POSTERIOR TIBIAL ARTERY

- It is the 2nd terminal branch formed at the bifurcation of popliteal artery at the lower level of popliteus.
- It passes underneath the fibrous arch of the soleus and courses

downwards on the tibialis posterior in between the flexor digitorum longus and flexor hallucis longus.

- Throughout its course, it is accompanied by a pair of venae comitantes.
- It terminates below the flexor retinaculum by dividing into its terminal branches.

***Branches***

1. Peroneal or fibular artery
2. Circumflex fibular artery
3. Medial plantar artery
4. Lateral plantar artery
5. Nutrient artery to tibia
6. Muscular arteries to flexor hallucis longus, flexor digitorum longus, tibialis posterior (deep flexors) and soleus

Pulsation of the posterior tibial artery can be palpated behind the medial malleolus, one inch from the medial border of tendocalcaneous. An arteriovenous shunt (fistula) of this artery with the great saphenous vein at this region is made by the surgeons for hemodialysis.

## VEINS OF THE LOWER LIMB

In the lower limbs, the veins are arranged in three groups.

### 1. Superficial Veins

This set of veins lies in the superficial fascia just beneath the skin. These veins consist of:

a. Great saphenous vein and its tributaries and

b. Small saphenous vein and its tributaries.

### 2. Deep Veins

These veins lie deep in the intermuscular septae or in between the muscle layers. These are:

a. Venae comitantes of the anterior tibial artery,

b. Venae comitantes of the posterior tibial artery,

c. Popliteal vein and tributaries and
d. Femoral vein and tributaries

### 3. Perforating Veins

These are the communicating vessels that connect the superficial and deep veins. They usually possess valves to prevent the retrograde flow of blood. These veins are found at the following sites:

a. Medial side of the leg
b. Ankle region

## Great or Long Saphenous Vein

### *Origin*

It begins as the continuation of the medial marginal vein (medial end of dorsal venous arch) of the foot. It is the longest vein of the body.

### *Course*

- From its origin, it courses upwards in front of medial malleolus.
- Here, it crosses the medial surface of the tibia in the lower part.
- It then ascends towards the knee behind the medial border of tibia behind the medial border of patella.
- It then takes a slight spiral course around the medial border of the thigh to come in front and upwards towards saphenous opening.

### *Termination*

It ends in the femoral vein in the saphenous opening through the cribriform fascia.

### Tributaries

#### *1. In the upper part*

a. Superficial circumflex iliac vein
b. Superficial epigastric vein
c. Superficial external pudendal vein
d. Deep external pudendal vein
e. Anterolateral vein of thigh
f. Posteromedial vein of thigh

g. A deep vein over adductor longus
h. A long perforator in the lower thigh

### *2. In the lower part*

a. A perforating vein just below the medial malleolus
b. A perforating vein 10 cm above the medial malleolus
c. A perforator in the middle or slightly lower in the leg
d. A perforator just below the knee
e. Posterior arch vein, a superficial longitudinal vein. All four perforators join this vein in the leg. The vein drains in the saphenous vein below the knee.
f. Venae comitantes of the posterior tibial artery
g. Venous plexus deep to soleus

> Great saphenous vein contains more than twenty valves to prevent the back flow of the blood against the gravity. Most of these valves are located in the segment of the vein which is below the knee. This vein was once very popular to be used in coronary arteries bypass operation.

## Tibiofibular Joints

### *1. Superior tibiofibular joint*

- It is a flat synovial joint.
- The articulating bones are head of fibula and the lateral condyle of the tibia.
- It is covered by the joint capsule.
- The anterior and posterior ligaments which are the thickened bands of the capsule provide stability to this joint.
- The joint cavity may communicate with the knee joint posteriorly through a bursa deep to the popliteus tendon.

### *2. Inferior tibiofibular joint*

- It is a fibrous joint of ***syndesmosis*** variety.
- The articulating bones are distal notch of tibia and distal end of fibula (medial surface).

- The ligaments which strongly hold the articulating bones together are:
    a. Anterior tibiofibular ligament
    b. Posterior tibiofibular ligament and
    c. Interosseous tibiofibular ligament.
- Only slight lateral rotation occurs at this joint during dorsiflexion of the foot.

## CLINICAL AND APPLIED INTEGRATION

### Soleal Pump (Peripheral Heart)

The soleus muscle contains a rich plexus of veins formed by the perforating veins of the great saphenous vein. The blood in these veins is pumped up against the gravity by the contraction of soleus muscle. The pumping action of the muscle aids the venous return and, therefore, is called peripheral heart. There is a danger of deep vein thrombosis due to prolonged pooling and stagnation of blood in these veins if this pump fails. The soleal pump is aided by the 'sole pump'. The veins of the plantar muscles of the sole of foot act as sole pump which pump most of the blood from sole into the dorsal venous arch of the foot.

The patients who become immobile due to paraplegia or hemiplegia or passangers travelling long distances and sitting immobile for hours are prone to deep vein thrombosis. If the thrombus is dislodged it may lead to pulmonary or coronary embolism which may become very fatal.

### Plantaris Tendon Autograft

This muscle is usually absent in 10% of population. It can be harvested for use in tendon graft. It is used as an autograft in the injuries to the flexor tendons of the fingers. Palmaris longus tendon is also being used by advanced surgeons in the same manner.

### Rupture of the Tendocalcaneous

Rupture of the tendocalcaneous is very common in athletes and tennis players. Active plantarflexion of the foot is lost. Patient feels sudden sharp pain and a gap at the site of insertion of the tendocalcaneous due to the retraction of gastrocnemius and soleus muscles.

## Venae Section (Venous Cut Down)

Venous cut down is usually performed as an emergency procedure for the transfusion of fluids and blood. When the commonly used veins of the upper limb collapse in shock or massive bleeding, venous cut down is indicated. Most commonly it is performed on the great saphenous vein. The site of cut down is infiltrated by the local anaesthesia to block the saphanous nerve and its branches in front of medial malleolus. A transverse incision is made through the skin and fascia just anterior and superior to the medial malleolus in the course of the vein. The vein is easily identified and a cannula or brannula is passed to establish the intravenous line.

## Varicose Veins

Prolonged stagnation or pooling of blood cause dilatation and tortuousity of the veins. Such veins are called as varicose veins and the condition as varicosity. Mostly veins of the leg are more affected. The important causes are the failure of soleal pump to empty the blood in the deep veins and the incompetent valves of the leg veins which work as antigravity factor. Prolonged sitting, standing, immobilization or blockage of the draining veins mays lead to varicosity.

Chapter

# 22 THE FOOT

**THE FOOT** bears the body weight and helps in propulsive movements. It also helps to balance the body in motion and in erect posture. The foot consists of:

1. Dorsum of the foot and
2. Sole of the foot.

## DORSUM OF THE FOOT

### Extensor Digitorum Brevis

#### *Origin*

1. Upper surface of the calcaneus
2. Inferior extensor retinaculum

#### *Insertion*

It gives off four tendons, one each for medial four toes.

- The tendon to the big toe separates from rest of the muscle and is inserted into the base of the proximal phalanx of the big toe.
- The other three tendons are inserted into the dorsal extensor expansions of the 2nd, 3rd and the 4th toe.

#### *Nerve supply*

Deep peroneal nerve

#### *Action*

It extends the medial four toes.

### Superior Extensor Retinaculum

It is the thickening of the deep fascia of the leg in front of the lower end of tibia.

### *Attachment*

- *Medially,* to the anterior border of the tibia
- *Laterally,* to the anterior border of the fibula

### *Structures passing beneath the retinaculum*

- *Tendons of* (from medial to lateral) tibialis anterior, extensor hallucis longus, extensor digitorum longus, peroneus tertius
- *Nerve,* deep peroneal nerve
- *Vessels,* anterior tibial artery and vein

## Inferior Extensor Retinaculum

It is a "Y" shaped thickening of the deep fascia of the leg, lying distal to the superior retinaculum on the dorsum of the foot.

### *Attachments*

- The stem of the retinaculum lies horizontally and is attached to the calcaneus.
- From the stem, two diverging limbs arise laterally. The upper one is attached to the medial malleolus. The lower limb crosses the medial longitudinal arch of the foot and merges with the plantar aponeurosis.

### *Structures passing beneath the retinaculum*

(Same as superior retinaculum)

- *Tendons of* (from medial to lateral) tibialis anterior, extensor hallucis longus, extensor digitorum longus, peroneus tertius
- *Nerve,* deep peroneal nerve
- *Vessels,* anterior tibial artery and vein

> The inferior extensor retinaculum prevents the bowstringing of the extensor tendons during their passage beneath the retinaculum towards the attachments.

## SUPERFICIAL PERONEAL (FIBULAR) NERVE

- It is one of the terminal branches of the common peroneal nerve.
- It begins in the substance of the peroneus longus.

- It courses in the distal third of the leg behind the anterior intermuscular septum.
- It divides into medial and lateral branches at the junction of middle and lower thirds.

### *Supply*

- Supplies the peroneus longus and brevis
- Skin on the anterolateral surface of the leg
- Skin of the dorsum of foot
- Medial side of the great toe
- Third and the fourth clefts

## Deep Peroneal Nerve

- It arises within peroneus longus over the neck of fibula.
- It spirals over the neck of the fibula to reach and course over the interosseus membrane.
- The anterior tibial vessels lie medial to it.
- It supplies the muscles of the extensor compartment (tibialis anterior, extensor hallucis longus, extensor digitorum longus and peroneus tertius).

## Dorsalis Pedis Artery

### *Origin*

It is the continuation of the anterior tibial artery (as its terminal branch) in the foot.

### *Course*

- It starts from the middle point between the medial and lateral malleoli lying over the lower end of the tibia.
- From here it extends forwards to the first intermetatarsal space.
- During its course on the dorsum of the foot, the tendon of extensor hallucis longus lies medial to it and digital branch of deep peroneal nerve laterally.
- The tendon of extensor hallucis brevis (which is the most medial tendinous slip of extensor digitorum brevis to the big toe) crosses it obliquely from lateral to medial on the dorsum of the foot.

- In the first intermetatarsal space, it dips down into the sole of the foot and joins the lateral plantar artery. The plantar arterial arch is thus completed by the union of the two vessels.

### *Termination*

It ends at the first intermetatarsal space.

### *Branches*

1. First dorsal metatarsal artery
2. Lateral tarsal artery
3. Arcuate artery

> *Pulsation* of dorsalis pedis artery can be felt between a line extending from the midpoint between the lateral and medial malleoli and the cleft of first toe.

## Dorsal Venous Arch

- It is formed over the heads of metatarsal bones.
- Its tributaries are:
  1. Medial marginal vein of the foot,
  2. Lateral marginal vein of the foot and
  3. Interosseous veins of the foot.
- Blood from its *medial end* is drained into the great saphenous vein.
- Blood from its *lateral end* is drained into the small saphenous vein.

# SOLE OF THE FOOT

## Plantar Aponeurosis

- It is the thickening of the deep fascia of the sole.
- It consists of longitudinally arranged dense collagenous fiber bundles lying underneath the skin of the sole.
- It is attached posteriorly to the calcaneus and fans out anteriorly.
- Anteriorly it divides into five slips, one for each toe.
- At the metatarsal bone heads its slips are connected with each other by *superficial transverse metatarsal ligament.*

- The five digital slips split to give way to the flexor tendons and are attached at the edges of *fibrous flexor sheath* and *deep transverse metatarsal ligaments.*
- From each edge of the plantar aponeurosis, a septum arises and is attached to the 1st and 5th metatarsal bones.
- It thus separates the abductors of the little and big toe from flexor digitorum brevis.
- It prevents the deeper structures in the sole from trauma.
- It also helps to maintain the bony arches of the foot, by acting as a tie beam.

## Muscles of the Sole of Foot

Muscles of the sole are arranged in four layers.

### 1. *Muscles of the first layer*

a. Abductor hallucis
b. Abductor digiti minimi
c. Flexor digitorum brevis

### 2. *Muscles of the second layer*

a. Tendon of flexor digitorum longus
b. Tendon of flexor hallucis longus
c. Flexor accessories
d. The lumbricles

### 3. *Muscles of the third layer*

a. Flexor hallucis brevis
b. Adductor hallucis
c. Flexor digiti minimi brevis

### 4. *Muscles of the fourth layer*

a. Dorsal and plantar interossei
b. Tendon of peroneus longus
c. Tendon of tibialis posterior

## Medial Plantar Artery

### *Origin*

- It is a terminal branch of the posterior tibial artery.
- It originates beneath the flexor retinaculum.

### *Termination*

It ends at the medial side of big toe.

### *Course*

It passes deep to flexor hallucis.

### *Branches*

1. Cutaneous branches
2. Muscular branches
3. Articular branches
4. Small superficial digital branches (three)

## Lateral Plantar Artery

### *Origin*

- It is the larger terminal branch of the posterior tibial artery.
- It originates beneath the flexor retinaculum.

### *Termination*

It ends at the base of fifth metatarsal bone.

### *Course*

It passes deep to abductor hallucis and then flexor digitorum brevis.

### *Branches*

1. Continues as plantar arch
2. Anastomotic
3. Occasionally branches to calcaneus

## Plantar Arch

### *Origin and formation*

- It is the continuation of the lateral plantar artery.
- It is completed by anastomosing with the dorsalis pedis artery.
- It extends from the base of fifth metatarsal bone to the first inter metatarsal space.

### *Location*

It lies in between the third and fourth layers of the sole.

### *Branches*

1. Plantar metatarsal artery (four). Each branch gives off:
    a. One distal perforating artery and
    b. Two plantar digital arteries.
2. Three perforating arteries (proximal)

## Medial Plantar Nerve

### *Origin*

- It is a terminal branch of the tibial nerve.
- It originates beneath the flexor retinaculum.

### *Termination*

It ends in between the abductor hallucis and flexor digitorum brevis.

### *Branches*

1. Cutaneous branch: Plantar digital nerve
2. Muscular branches: Abductor hallucis, flexor digitorum brevis, flexor hallucis brevis, first lumbrical
3. Articular branches: To small joint of foot

## Lateral Plantar Nerve

### *Origin*

- It is a terminal branch of the tibial nerve.
- It originates beneath the flexor retinaculum.

### *Termination*

It ends at the base of fifth metatarsal bone.

### *Branches*

1. Muscular branches: Quadratus plantae, abductor digiti minimi
2. Terminal branches: a. Superficial branch b. Deep branch

## ANKLE JOINT

- It is a synovial joint of modified hinge variety.
- Articulating bony surfaces are inferior facet of the tibia, upper facet of the talus, medial and lateral malleoli.
- Joint capsule is attached to the margins of all the articulating bones except the front of talus.
- Synovial membrane lines the inner side of the capsule and is attached to the articular margins.

### Ligaments of the Ankle Joint

1. Deltoid ligament
2. Lateral ligament
3. Anterior talofibular ligament
4. Posterior talofibular ligament
5. Calcaneofibular ligament
6. Posterior tibiofibular ligament
7. Inferior transverse ligament

### Movements at Ankle Joint

#### *Dorsiflexion (10°)*

- Tibialis anterior
- Extensor hallucis longus
- Extensor digitorum longus
- Peroneus tertius

#### *Plantarflexion (20°)*

- Gastrocnemius

- Soleus
- Assisted by flexor digitorum longus, peroneus longus and peroneus brevis

The strongest ligament of the ankle joint is the deltoid ligament. The weak ligaments which are usually ruptured by injury are anterior talofibular and calcaneofibular ligaments.

## Subtalar Joint

- It is a synovial joint of plane variety.
- Articulation occurs between the inferior surface of the body of talus and the facet on the upper surface of calcaneus on the posterior parts.
- Joint is enclosed by a capsule which is attached to the margins of the articular surfaces.
- Synovial membrane lines the capsule.
- Ligaments:
  1. Medial talocalcaneal ligament
  2. Lateral talocalcaneal ligament
  3. Interosseous ligament (attached above to sulcus tali and below to sulcus calcanei)

## Midtarsal Joint

This joint is a combination of two small joints of the tarsal bones:

### *1. Talocalcaneonavicular joint*

- It is the anterior joint between talus and calcaneum along with the navicular bone.
- It is also of synovial variety and is incompletely enclosed by the capsule.
- Ligament: Plantar calcaneonavicular ligament
- Gliding and rotator movements occur at this joint.

### *2. Calcaneocuboid joint*

- It is a synovial joint of plane variety, enclosed in the capsule.

- It is an articulation between the anterior end of the calcaneus and the posterior surface of the cuboid.
- Ligaments:
  a. Bifurcated (Y-shaped) ligament
  b. Long plantar ligament
  c. Short plantar ligament

## MOVEMENTS AT SUBTALAR AND MIDTARSAL JOINTS

### 1. Inversion of the Foot

- It is the movement when the sole of the foot moves inwards and the medial border of the foot is raised off the ground.
- It occurs on the subtalar and subtarsal joints.
- Muscles producing this movement are tibialis anterior, tibialis posterior, assisted by flexor and extensor hallucis longus.
- The range of movement during inversion is increased in plantarflexion.

### 2. Eversion of the Foot

- It is the movement when the sole of the foot faces outwards and the lateral border of the foot is raised off the ground.
- It occurs on the subtalar and subtarsal joints.
- Muscles producing this movement are peroneus longus, peroneus brevis and peroneus tertius.
- The range of movement during inversion is increased in dorsiflexion.

## ARCHES OF THE FOOT

The arches of the foot provide stability to human body in the erect as well as mobile posture by inculcating the following factors:

1. Distribution of body weight on to the feet
2. Acting as shock absorbers to cope with the impacts transmitted e.g. when landing on the ground
3. Providing a spring action for walking and jumping mechanisms

4. Providing resilience to the feet so that it can adapt to the changes while moving on smooth, even or irregular surfaces

The weight of the body is supported on the following three arches of each foot:

a. Medial longitudinal arch

b. Lateral longitudinal arch

c. Transverse arch

## a. Medial Longitudinal Arch

### *Formation*

- Calcaneums
- Talus
- Navicular
- Medial, intermediate and lateral cuneiform bones
- Medial three (1st, 2nd and 3rd) metatarsals

### *Keystone*

Head of the talus

## Maintenance of the Medial Longitudinal Arch

### *Configuration of the tarsal bones*

- The sustentaculum tali (a bony projection on the medial side of calcaneus) supports the talus medially.
- The concave upper surface of navicular bone holds the head of talus.
- The medial cuneiform supports the navicular bone.

### *Tie beams or bowstrings (Horizontal supports)*

- Plantar aponeurosis
- Spring ligament
- *Tendons*: Flexor hallucis longus, flexor digitorum longus
- *Muscles of first layer of sole:* Abductor hallucis and medial half of flexor digitorum brevis

### *Interlocking ligaments and enforcement ties*

- Plantar calcaneonavicular ligament
- Tibialis posterior insertions

### *Suspension supports (Vertical supports)*

- *Medially:* Tibialis anterior tendon
- *Laterally:* Peroneus longus tendon

## b. Lateral Longitudinal Arch

### *Formation*

- Calcaneus
- Cuboid
- Lateral two ($4^{th}$ and $5^{th}$) metatarsals

### *Keystone*

Cuboid

## Maintenance of the Lateral Longitudinal Arch

### *Configuration of the tarsal bones*

- Bony factors play no role in the maintenance of this arch.

### *Tie beams or bowstrings (Horizontal supports)*

- Plantar aponeurosis
- Short and long plantar ligaments
- *Tendons*: Flexor digitorum longus
- *Muscles of first layer of sole:* Abductor digiti minimi and lateral half of flexor digitorum brevis

### *Interlocking ligaments and enforcement ties*

- Plantar calcaneonavicular ligament
- Tibialis posterior insertions

### *Suspension supports (Vertical supports)*

- Peroneus longus tendon

## c. Transverse Arch

*Formation*

- Bases of all five metatarsals
- Cuboid
- Medial, intermediate and lateral cuneiform bones

## Maintenance of the Transverse Arch

*Configuration of the tarsal bones*

- The wedge shape of intermediate and lateral cuneiform bones
- Cuboid to some extent

*Tie beams or bowstrings (Horizontal supports)*

- Peroneus longus tendon

*Interlocking ligaments and enforcement ties*

- Deep transverse ligament
- Plantar ligaments
- Dorsal interossei and transverse head of abductor hallucis

*Suspension supports (Vertical supports)*

- Peroneus longus tendon
- Peroneus brevis tendon

## CLINICAL AND APPLIED INTEGRATION

## Compartmental Syndrome

The compression of the extensor compartment of the leg by oedema, hematoma, or any space occupying lesion or tumour may lead to the loss of blood supply (ischemia) to its contents. This condition is known as compartmental syndrome. The extensor compartment of the leg is a space between the deep fascia (anteriorly), Interosseous membrane (posteriorly), extensor surface of tibia (medially), extensor surface of fibula and anterior intermuscular septum (laterally).

The contents of extensor compartment are:

1. Muscles: Tibialis anterior, extensor hallucis longus, extensor digitorum longus, peroneus tertius

2. Nerves: Deep peroneal nerve
3. Vessels: Anterior tibial artery and vein

## Genu Valgum

The lateral angulation of the leg in relation to the thigh in which Q-angle is large (>17°) is called genu valgum. It is also called as knock-knee.

## Genu Varum

The medial angulation of the leg in relation to the thigh in which Q-angle is small is called genu varum deformity. In this condition, the femur is abnormally vertical. The line bearing weight falls medial to the center of the knee.

## Pes Planus (Flat Foot)

It is characterized by the complete or partial absence of bony arches of the foot. It is of two types

1. *Flexible flat foot* when it is conspicous on weight bearing and is not visible normally. The medial longitudinal arch is usually at fault in this verity of flat foot.
2. *Rigid flat foot* which is obvious even when the foot is not bearing weight.

Flat foot may be acquired when it is secondary to the dysfunction of tibialis posterior. The arches of the foot are collapsed due to trauma or any age-related degeneration.

Chapter

# 23 MISCELLANEOUS

## RADIOGRAPHS OF THE LOWER LIMB

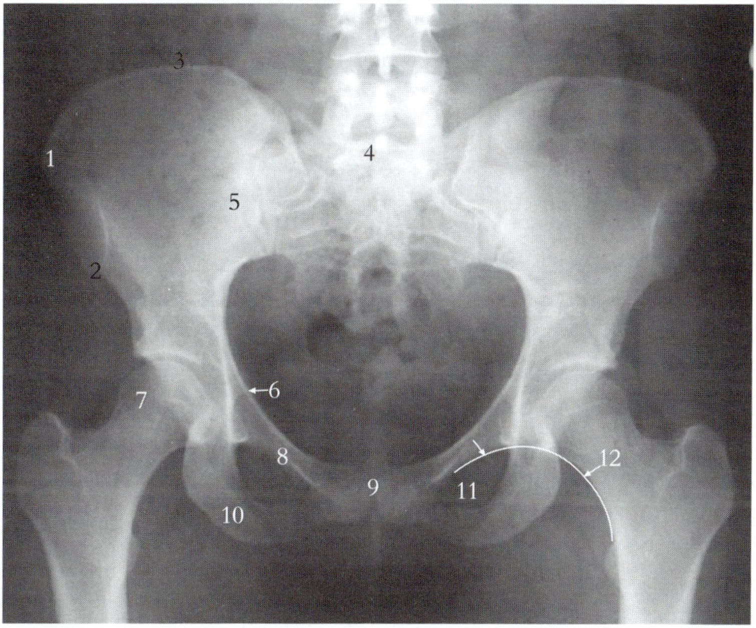


Fig. 23.1: X-ray of adult pelvis (AP view)

1. Anterior superior iliac spine 2. Anterior inferior iliac spine 3. Iliac crest 4. Promontory 5. Sacro-iliac joint 6. Ischial spine 7. Head of femur 8. Superior pubic ramus 9. Pubic symphysis 10. Inferior ramus of pubis 11. Obturator foramen 12. Shenton's line

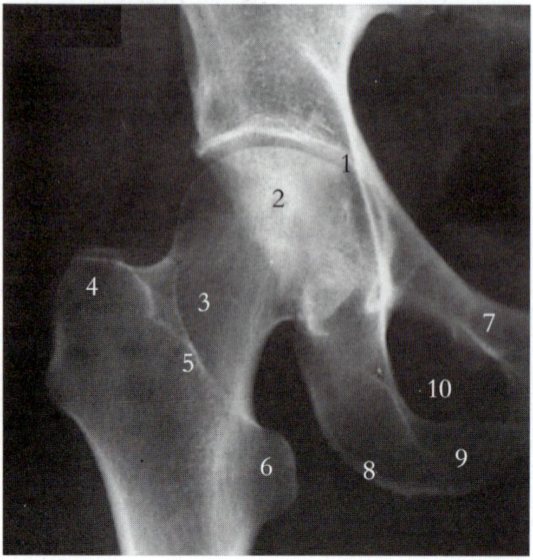


**Fig. 23.2: X-ray of hip joint (AP view) showing the bony landmarks of articulating bones**

1. Acetabulum 2. Head of femur 3. Neck of femur 4. Greater trochanter of femur 5. Intertrochanteric line 6. Lesser trochanter of femur 7. Superior ramus of pubis 8. Ischial tuberosity 9. Inferior ramus of pubis 10. Obturator foramen

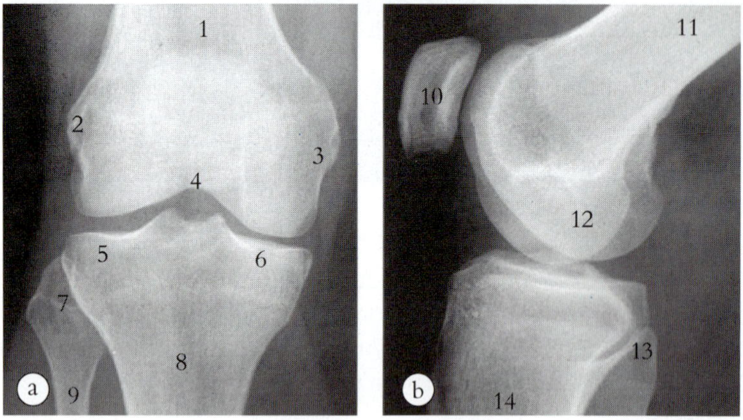


**Fig. 23.3: X-ray of knee joint (a) AP view (b) lateral view, showing the bony landmarks of articulating bones**

1. Femur 2. Lateral epicondyle of femur 3. Medial epicondyle of femur 4. Intercondylar fossa 5. Lateral condyle of tibia 6. Medial condyle of

tibia 7. Head of fibula 8. Tuberosity of tibia 9. Fibula neck 10. Patella 11. Shaft of femur 12. Lateral condyle of femur 13. Styloid process of fibula 14. Tibia

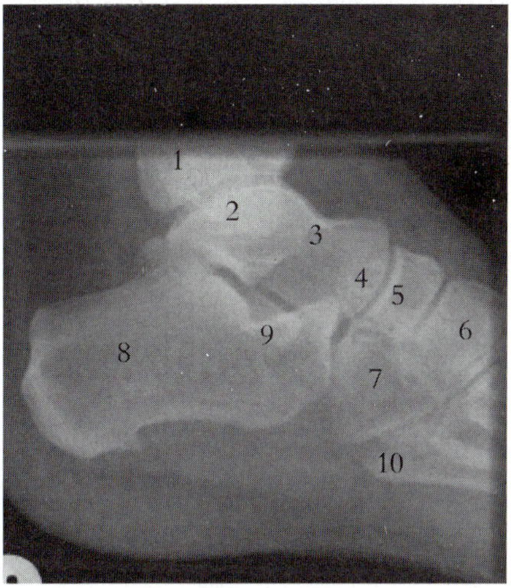


**Fig. 23.4: X-ray of ankle joint (lateral view) showing the tarsal bones**

1. Tibia 2. Talus 3. Neck of talus 4. Head of talus 5. Navicular 6. Lateral cuneiform 7. Cuboid 8. Calcaneus 9. Sustentaculum tali 10. Fifth metatarsal

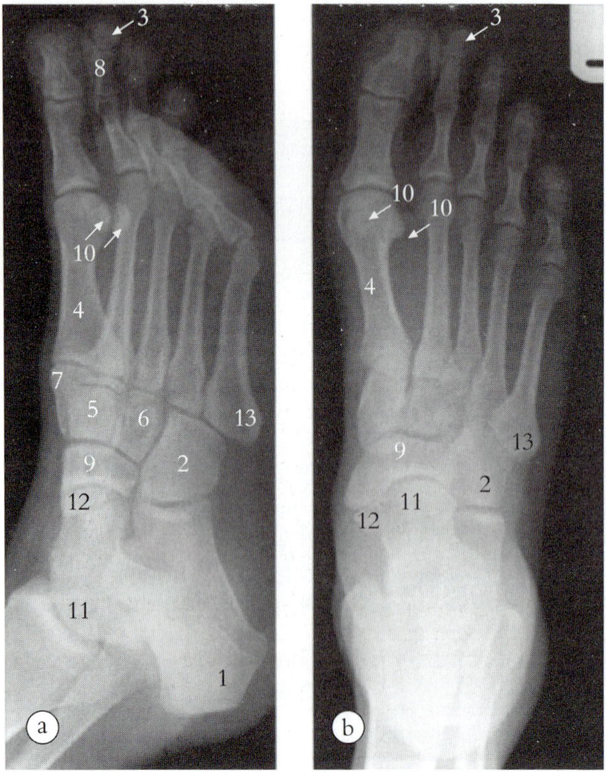


**Fig. 23.5: X-ray of foot showing (a) lateral view (b) dorsal view**

1. Calcaneus 2. Cuboid 3. Distal phalanx of second toe 4. First metatarsal 5. Intermediate cuneiform 6. Lateral cuneiform 7. Medial cuneiform 8. Middle phalanx of second toe 9. Navicular 10. Sesamoid bones in flexor hallucis brevis muscles 11. Talus 12. Navicular bone

## COMMON SITES OF FRACTURES AND DISLOCATIONS OF LOWER LIMB WITH THE RELATED NERVE INJURY

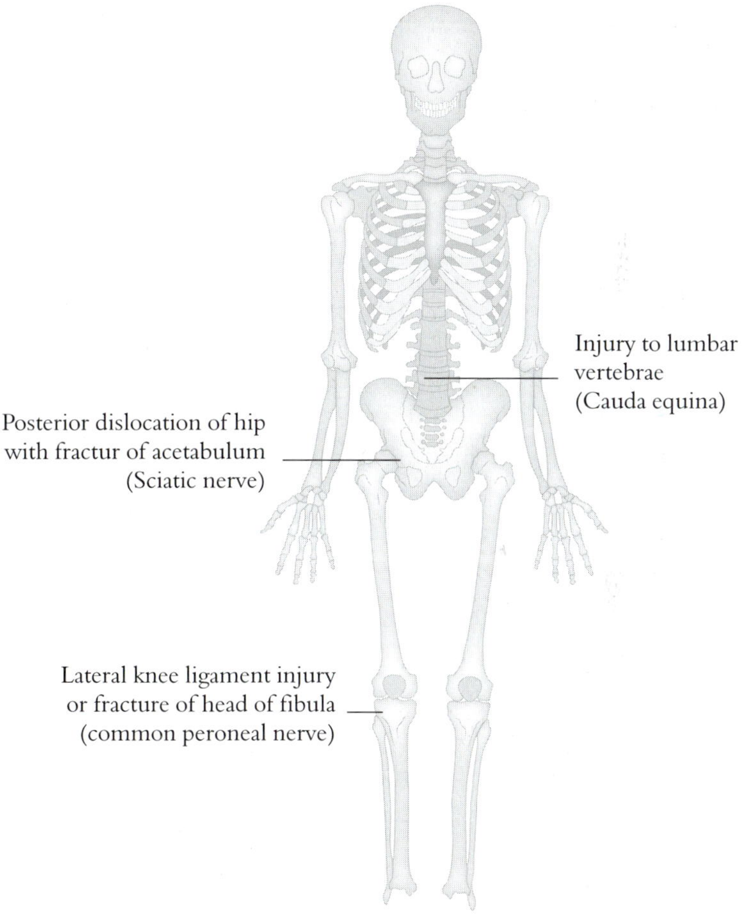


**Fig. 23.6: Schematic diagram showing the common side of fracture and nerve injury of lower limb**

## SURFACE ANATOMY

### Femoral Artery

It lies on the upper two-thirds of a line drawn between the following points (with the thigh in a position of slight flexion, abduction and lateral rotation).

1. Mid-inguinal point
2. Adductor tubercle

### Profunda Femoris Artery

Joins the two points deep to the course of femoral artery:

1. Below 3.5 cm of mid-inguinal point
2. Below 10 cm of mid-inguinal point

### Popliteal Artery

It lies at the back of the lower 1/3$^{rd}$ of thigh and upper 1/3$^{rd}$ of leg extending between the:

1. 2.5 cm medial to the middle on the back of lower 1/3$^{rd}$ of thigh
2. Middle of the back of knee
3. On the tibial tuberosity

### Superior Gluteal Artery

It lies posteriorly on the upper 1/3$^{rd}$ of a line joining the:

1. Posterior superior iliac spine and
2. Apex of the greater trochanter.

### Anterior Tibial Artery

Joins the points between:

1. Half inch below the medial side of fibula and
2. Middle of two malleoli.

### Posterior Tibial Artery

It lies on the line joining the points at the following locations:

1. On the tibial tuberosity (at the back of leg)
2. Middle of the medial malleolus and tendocalcaneous

## Dorsalis Pedis Artery

Joins a line at the following points:

1. Middle of two malleoli
2. At the proximal end of the first intermetatarsal space

## Plantar Arch

It lies between the following two points:

1. 2.5 cm medial to the tuberosity of $5^{th}$ metatarsal
2. In the first intermetatarsal space, 2.5 cm distal to the tuberosity of navicular bone

## Femoral Vein

It lies on a line joining the following points:

1. 1 cm medial to the mid-inguinal point
2. 1 cm lateral to the adductor tubercle

## Great Saphenous Vein

It is a long vein marked by joining the following points.

1. Medial end of dorsal venous arch (on the dorsum of foot)
2. Anterior to medial malleolus
3. The junction of middle and lower third of the medial border of the tibia
4. Adductor tubercle
5. 3 cm below and lateral to the pubic tubercle, (i.e. at the saphenous opening)

## Small Saphenous Vein

It lies on a line joining the following points.

1. Lateral end of dorsal venous arch
2. Posterior to lateral malleolus
3. Middle of popliteal fossa

## Femoral Nerve

It is marked on the points joining the following locations:

1. Lateral to the mid-inguinal point (1.5 cm)
2. Then 2.5 cm below this point

## Sciatic Nerve

It lies deeply to the gluteal region. It is marked by joining the following points:

1. Mid-point between ischeal tuberosity and greater trochanter
2. Apex of popliteal fossa

## Tibial Nerve

It lies on a line joining the points between:

1. Apex of popliteal fossa (at the lower third of back of thigh),
2. Tibial tuberosity and
3. Between the medial malleolus and tendocalcaneous.

## Common Peroneal Nerve

It lies on a line joining the:

1. Apex of politeal fossa and
2. Back of the neck of fibula.

## Deep Peroneal Nerve

It is marked by a line between the:

1. Neck of the fibula and
2. Center of the line joining the two malleoli anteriorly.

## Inguinal Ligament

It stretches with a slight downward convexity between the:

1. Anterior superior iliac spine and
2. Pubic tubercle.

## Saphenous Opening

1. Take a point 3 cm below the pubic tubercle and draw a line horizontally from this point.
2. Now take another point 3 cm lateral to the pubic tubercle and draw a vertical line.
3. Saphenous opening lies at the intersection of the horizontal and vertical lines.

Chapter

# 24 SEQs

1. Draw and label a diagram of popliteal fossa showing its boundaries and contents.
2. Name the ligaments and nerves of the ankle joint. Which ligament is the strongest and which of them are usually injured in such cases?
3. Name the muscles of first layer of sole of foot. Write the area of cutaneous sensory loss and muscles paralysed in case of injury to the medial plantar nerve.
4. Write the location and arrangement of superficial inguinal lymph nodes. Mention areas of lymph drainage by afferent lymph vessels of these lymph nodes and destination of their efferent vessels.
5. a. Write the origin and course of profunda femoris artery.
   b. Name its branches. Which of these branches are the main source of blood supply to the head and neck of the femur?
6. Medical students were being demonstrated ankle jerk reflex. Which anatomical structure is utilized to elicit this reflex? Write the formation and attachment of this structure and the nerves put to test this reflex. What is the result of ankle jerk reflex if these nerves are injured?
7. a. Write the arterial supply of knee joint.
   b. Which of these arteries will supply the intra-articular structures of knee joint and how will it reach them? What is the clinical importance of this profuse arterial supply?
8. a. Name the ligaments located deep to gluteus maximus and mention their attachments.
   b. List the nerves and vessels passing through the greater sciatic foramen.
9. a. Name the articulating surfaces of ankle joint.
   b. Write a brief account of structures binding them together.

10. Write the formation and anatomical location of two arterial anastomosis of gluteal region. Mention their functions.
11. Write formation of femoral sheath and give the anatomical reason why femoral nerve is not within the femoral sheath? Why femoral hernia is more liable to strangulation?
12. Write origin, course, relations and mode of termination and branches of posterior tibial artery. How posterior tibial pulse is palpated?
13. Give the attachment, nerve supply and actions of muscles attached to medial surface of tibia in a tabulated form.
14. List six structures passing underneath the superior extensor retinaculum at lower region of leg. Explain functionally "too long" lower limb. Mention three causes of too long lower limb. Explain three means of compensation for this problem during walking.
15. List two causes of injury to common peroneal nerve. Mention the motor and sensory deficits as well as 'gait' of such a person.

# INDEX


**A**

Adductor canal 155, 156, 160
Anastomosis
  around elbow joint 108
  around knee joint 181
  arterial anastomosis 67, 224
  arteriovenous 196
  cruciate 167
  end-to-end 36
  scapular 67, 68
  transverse 36, 67, 169
  trochanteric 169
Anatomical planes
  axial 6
  coronal 6, 7
  frontal 6
  median 6, 7
  midsagittal 5
  sagittal 6, 7
  transverse or horizontal 6
Anatomical snuffbox 118
Anatomical terms 6
  laterality 8
  positions 6
Anatomy 3, 4
  applied 4
  comparative 4
  embryology or developmental 3
  general 3
  gross anatomy 3
  histology or microanatomy 3
  investigative 4
  physiological or functional 4
  radiological 4
  regional 17, 42
  surface 3, 11, 18
  systemic 3, 37
Angiography 52
Aponeurosis
  palmar aponeurosis 128, 134, 136, 138, 147
  plantar 204, 205, 206, 207
Arches of the foot 210
  lateral longitudinal arch 212
  medial longitudinal arch 211, 213
  transverse arch 213
Arteries 33
  anterior tibial 195, 196, 202, 203, 214
  axillary 35, 57, 63
  brachial 44, 57, 58
  dorsalis pedis 204, 207
  femoral 33, 151, 152, 155
  lateral circumflex femoral 169
  plantar 154, 183, 196
  popliteal 35, 152, 160
  posterior tibial 182, 196, 198, 206, 224
  profunda brachii 108
  radial 33, 36, 69, 99
  subclavian 33, 35, 58, 67, 68

ulnar 33, 36, 70, 91
Arterioles 33
Atherosclerosis 37
Avascular necrosis 169
Axilla 55, 81, 87
Axillary sheath 85
Axillary tail 92, 94, 96

**B**

Baker's cyst 189
Bone
age assessment 20
appendicular 25, 57
axial 25, 26, 27
blood supply 27, 37, 128, 163, 164, 169
cartilaginous 15
compact (haversian) 13
membrano-cartilaginous 15
membranous 94, 151
pneumatic 15
spongy (cancellous) 13
Breast 96
Bronchoscopy 49
Bursa
ansarina 188
subacromial (subdeltoid) 75

**C**

Canal of guyon 129
Capillaries
continuous 23, 128, 130, 134, 151
fenestrated 34
sinusoidal 36
Carpal tunnel 148
Carrying angle 106
Cartilages 18
elastic 33, 35, 36
fibrocartilage 30, 31, 66, 127
hyaline 30, 31, 66, 124
Cervicoaxillary canal 82
Cleavage lines 11
Coxa valga 177
Ct scan 51, 52
Cystoscopy 50

**D**

Deep vein thrombosis 199
Dermatomes of
lower limb 155, 158, 159, 191
upper limb 68, 69, 81, 83, 86, 89, 91, 99, 111, 127
Development
postnatal 4
prenatal 4
Dorsal venous arch 36
Dupuytren's contracture 147

**E**

Endoscopy 49
Endoskeleton 15
Exoskeleton 15

**F**

Facial palsy 27
Fascia
axillary 63, 67, 68
cervical 67
clavipectoral 62
cribriform 151, 152
lata 151, 152
scarpa 152
Felon 138
Femoral
artery catheterization 164
canal 155, 156, 157
hernia 158, 163, 164
pulse 164
sheath 156, 157, 158, 159

triangle 155, 159
Fibrous flexor sheath 130, 205
Flexor lines 11
Foot
arches 210, 211, 214
dorsum 202, 203
sole 204, 205
Foramen
greater sciatic 168, 223
lesser sciatic 166, 168
Fossa
cubital 104, 105
popliteal 179, 180
Fracture
bennett's 138
compound 184
green stick 19
simple 97
spontaneous 19
Frozen shoulder 79

**G**

Ganglia
parasympathetic 46
paravertebral 45, 46
prevertebral 45, 46, 85
sensory 39
sympathetic 91
Gastroscopy 49
Genu valgum (knock knee) 188
Genu varum (bow knee) 188
Glenoid labrum 78, 176
Golfer's elbow 109
Grip 137
Guy ropes 101
Gynaecomastia 97

**H**

Haemodialysis 196
Hemiplegia 27, 199
Holden's line 152
Housemaid's knee 189
Hypothenar eminence 133

**I**

Iliotibial tract 153
Interosseous membrane 112, 113, 191, 192, 194, 213

**J**

Joints
acromioclavicular 57
ankle 30
biaxial 30, 127
bicondylar 30
calcaneocuboid 209
cartilaginous 15
complex joints 30
compound 184
diarthroses 29
dislocation 32
elbow 30
ellipsoid 30
fibrous 29, 30
gomphoses 29
hilton's law 53
hinge 30
hip 30, 32
knee 30, 31, 32, 188
midtarsal 209
multiaxial 173
pivot joints 30
plane 30
radioulnar 30, 31, 117, 127
sellar or saddle 30
shoulder 29, 30, 32
simple joints 29
spheroidal 30

sternoclavicular 30, 57, 66
subtalar 210
sutural 29
symphyses 29
synarthroses 29
synchondroses 29
syndemoses 29
synovial joints 30, 32, 53, 54
talocalcaneonavicular 209
tibiofibular 195, 198, 199, 208
uniaxial 54
wrist 30

## L

Labra 31
Laparoscopy 49
Layers of skin
dermis 11, 94
epidermis 9
hypodermis 9, 24
Ligaments
costoclavicular 66
costocoracoid 62
deep transverse metatarsal 205
inguinal 220, 221, 223
intracapsular 182
lacunar 157, 158, 163
of ankle 191, 192, 194, 195, 217, 223
of cooper 94
posterior cruciate 185
radial (lateral) collateral 106
superficial transverse metatarsal 204
ulnar (medial) collateral 105
Lumpectomy 97
Lymph nodes
axillary 92, 93
pectoral region 3, 92
Lymphoid organs 38
Lymph vessels
afferent 38
efferent 38

## M

Magnetic resonance imaging (mri) 52
Mallet finger 138
Mammogram 142
Mastectomy 97
Mechanism of
abduction 7, 76, 77, 128, 131, 166, 175
unlocking of the knee 188
Menisci 19, 31, 185, 187
Metarterioles 33, 35
Miner's knee 189
Movements of
ankle 30
elbow joint 30
hip joint 30, 32
knee joint 30, 31
radioulnar joint 30, 125
scapula 57, 58, 59, 60, 64, 67, 68, 70, 71, 73, 74, 77, 82, 90, 139, 148
subtalar joint 209
thumb 8, 69, 70, 113, 116, 118, 127, 130, 131, 135, 136, 137, 138, 141, 148
wrist joint 30
Muscle contraction
isometric 23
isotonic 23
phasic 23
reflex 223
tonic 23
Muscle fibre
fast 24
intermediate 24
red 24

slow 21, 24
white 24
Muscles
antagonist 23
appendicular 25
axial 25, 26, 27
biceps brachii 22, 76
boxer's muscle 60
brachialis 88, 102, 120, 121
cardiac 24
climbing muscle 62
coracobrachialis 102
deltoid 22, 69, 71
extensor digitorum brevis 203
fixators 23
gluteus maximus 153, 173, 177, 223
gluteus medius 177
gluteus minimus 177
infraspinatus 73, 74
interossei 22, 134, 136, 148, 205, 213
involuntary 27, 45
latissimus dorsi 22, 82
levator scapulae 60, 64, 88
lumbricals 123, 124, 133, 136, 137
paralysis 27, 70, 73, 91, 148, 177
paresis 27
parts 3, 5, 33, 83, 113, 135, 209
pectoralis major 69, 82
pectoralis minor 62, 63, 83, 92
plantaris 179, 180, 187, 191
popliteus 180, 186, 187, 188, 195, 198
quadriceps femoris 185
rhomboid major 59, 63, 64
rhomboid minor 59, 63
serratus anterior 70, 90
skeletal 23, 24, 26, 27, 43, 44, 53
smooth 11, 16, 25, 33, 34, 44, 211
somatic 44, 45
spasm 80
subclavius 62, 63, 88, 90
subscapularis 22, 74, 89
supraspinatus 75, 78, 79, 80
synergists 23
tensor fascia lata 153, 175
teres major 83, 85, 107
teres minor 65, 73, 103
trapezius 71
triceps 65, 89, 101, 102, 108, 109, 120, 121
visceral 10, 44, 45
voluntary 23

## N

Nerves
axillary 69, 71, 79
common peroneal (fibular) 184
cranial 44, 46
cutaneous 69, 167
deep peroneal 202, 203, 214
femoral 167, 169, 171, 174, 175
functional components 44
intercostals 64, 82, 95, 96
lateral plantar 204, 207
medial plantar 223
median 6, 7, 70, 85, 88, 113, 119, 123, 124, 127, 129, 130, 133, 137, 138
musculocutaneous 103, 124
of bell 90
phrenic 96
radial 69
sciatic 162, 166, 168, 173, 175, 176, 177, 180
spinal 41, 42, 43, 44, 46, 53, 86, 173
splanchnic 46, 172
superficial peroneal 154, 184, 194

ulnar 70
Nervous system
autonomic 21, 43, 44, 45, 46
central 17, 41, 44, 87, 130, 135
peripheral 35, 199
Neuroglia 41
Neuron
afferent 26, 33, 38, 43, 223
bipolar 41
efferent 26, 33, 38, 43, 93, 223
interneurons 41
multipolar 41
parts 3, 5, 33, 83, 113, 135, 209
unipolar 41

**O**

Osteoarthritis 32
Osteomalacia 19
Osteomyelitis 20
Osteoporosis 19

**P**

Painful arc syndrome 80
Palmar arch 134, 135
Paralysis
crutch 91
erb's (duchenne) 90
gluteus maximus 153, 173, 177, 223
klumpke's 91, 148
saturday night 91
Paraplegia 27, 199
Pes planus (flat foot) 214
Plexus
brachial 87, 89, 90, 91
lumbar 42, 44, 62, 160, 170
sacral 42, 44, 172, 173
subsartorial 163
Preferential 33
Proctoscopy 50
Protoplasm 4

**Q**

Quadriplegia 27

**R**

Radial (humeral) groove 101
Radiograph
adult pelvis 215
ankle joint 217, 223
elbow joint 140
foot 218
hand and wrist 141
hip joint 216
knee joint 216
shoulder 139
Receptors
exteroceptive 44
interoceptive 44
proprioceptive 44, 137
teleceptors 45
Retinacular fibres 169, 174
Retinaculum
extensor 117
flexor 128, 129
inferior extensor 201
superior extensor 224
Rickets 19
Rotator cuff 79

**S**

Saphenous opening 222
Sciatica 177
Shenton's line 177, 215
Shunts 36
Sleeping foot 173
Soleal pump 199
Sole pump 199
Spaces
lower triangular 107

of parona 148
palmar 136, 138
pulp 137, 138
quadangular 103
reteromammary 97
upper triangular 65
web 136
Sprains 11
Student's elbow 109
Surface anatomy
anterior tibial artery 195, 196, 202, 203, 214
axillary artery 144
axillary nerve 145
brachial artery 144
common peroneal nerve 170, 189, 202, 224
deep palmar arch 144
deep peroneal nerve 202, 203, 214
dorsalis pedis artery 204, 207
extensor retinaculum 146
femoral artery 156, 157, 161, 164, 169, 174, 180, 182, 220
femoral nerve 151, 159, 188, 224
femoral vein 156, 157, 158, 159, 160, 182
flexor retinaculum 146
great saphenous vein 27, 152, 156, 196, 199, 200, 204
inguinal ligament 152, 156, 157, 158, 159, 160, 161, 164
median nerve 70, 85, 88, 113, 119, 123, 127, 129, 130, 133, 138
musculocutaneous nerve 103
plantar arch 206
popliteal artery 160, 161, 180, 182, 195
posterior tibial artery 196, 198, 206, 224
profunda femoris artery 161, 169, 223
radial 144
radial nerve 145
saphenous opening 151, 152, 157, 197, 221
sciatic nerve 151, 162, 173, 176, 177, 180, 183, 184, 188
small saphenous vein 27, 204
superficial palmar arch 144
superior gluteal artery 169
tibial nerve 170, 180, 182, 207
ulnar artery 144
ulnar nerve 145
Synovial fluid 32
Synovial sheath 10

## T

Tendocalcaneous 199
Tendon 10, 99, 105, 128, 166, 168, 199, 205
Tension lines 11
Thenar eminence 130
Thoracic duct 93
Trendelenburg test 177
Triangle
lumbar 42, 44, 62, 160, 170
of auscultation 107
Tubercles of montgomery 94

## U

Ultrasonography 51

## V

Varicosity 37, 200
Veins
axillary 35
femoral 156, 157
great saphenous 35, 152, 156
large 34
medium 33, 35

of the lower limb 34, 37, 151, 153, 155, 159
of upper limb 54, 57, 91, 99, 111, 143
popliteal 35
small 34, 35, 36
varicose 200
Venae comitantes 35, 85, 99, 196, 198
Venae section 200
Venules
collecting 34
muscular 17, 21, 34, 35, 36, 57, 65
postcapillary 34, 35
Vessel
capacitance 35
conducting 33
distribution 13, 173, 177
exchange 34, 35
resistance 33, 35

**W**

Waddling gait 177
Winging of scapula 148
Witch's milk 95